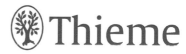

Pseudophakic Monovision

A Clinical Guide

Fuxiang Zhang, MD
Medical Director
Downriver Optimeyes Supervision Center
Senior Staff
Department of Ophthalmology
Henry Ford Health System
Taylor, Michigan

Alan Sugar, MD
Professor
Vice Chair
Ophthalmology and Visual Sciences
Kellogg Eye Center
University of Michigan
Ann Arbor, Michigan

Graham D. Barrett, MB, BCh, SAf, FRACO, FRACS
Clinical Professor
The University of Western Australia
Perth, Australia
Consultant Ophthalmic Surgeon
Lions Eye Institute
Consultant Ophthalmic Surgeon
Sir Charles Gardiner Hospital
Nedlands, Australia

49 illustrations

Thieme
New York • Stuttgart • Delhi • Rio de Janeiro

Executive Editor: William Lamsback
Managing Editor: Elizabeth Palumbo
Director, Editorial Services: Mary Jo Casey
Assistant Managing Editor: Haley Paskalides
Production Editor: Naamah Schwartz
International Production Director: Andreas Schabert
Editorial Director: Sue Hodgson
International Marketing Director: Fiona Henderson
International Sales Director: Louisa Turrell
Director of Institutional Sales: Adam Bernacki
Senior Vice President and Chief Operating Officer:
  Sarah Vanderbilt
President: Brian D. Scanlan

Library of Congress Cataloging-in-Publication Data
Names: Zhang, Fuxiang, MD, author. | Sugar, Alan, author. |
Barrett, Graham, (Ophthalmologist), author.
Title: Pseudophakic monovision / Fuxiang Zhang, Alan Sugar,
  Graham Barrett.
Description: New York : Thieme, [2019] |
Identifiers: LCCN 2018005469 (print) | LCCN 2018006724
  (ebook) | ISBN 9781626238947 (e-book) | ISBN
  9781626238930 (print)
Subjects: | MESH: Lens Implantation, Intraocular | Visual
  Acuity–physiology | Presbyopia–surgery | Pseudophakia–
  surgery
Classification: LCC RE938.5 (ebook) | LCC RE938.5 (print) |
  NLM WW 260 | DDC
  617.7/55–dc23
LC record available at https://lccn.loc.gov/2018005469

© 2019 Thieme Medical Publishers, Inc.

Thieme Publishers New York
333 Seventh Avenue, New York, NY 10001 USA
+1 800 782 3488, customerservice@thieme.com

Thieme Publishers Stuttgart
Rüdigerstrasse 14, 70469 Stuttgart, Germany
+49 [0]711 8931 421, customerservice@thieme.de

Thieme Publishers Delhi
A-12, Second Floor, Sector-2, Noida-201301
Uttar Pradesh, India
+91 120 45 566 00, customerservice@thieme.in

Thieme Publishers Rio de Janeiro, Thieme Publicações Ltda.
Edifício Rodolpho de Paoli, 25º andar
Av. Nilo Peçanha, 50 – Sala 2508
Rio de Janeiro 20020-906 Brasil
+55 21 3172-2297 / +55 21 3172-1896

Cover design: Thieme Publishing Group
Typesetting by Thomson Digital, India

Printed in The United States of America by King Printing
Company, Inc.   5 4 3 2 1

ISBN 978-1-62623-893-0

Also available as an e-book:
eISBN 978-1-62623-894-7

Important note: Medicine is an ever-changing science undergoing continual development. Research and clinical experience are continually expanding our knowledge, in particular our knowledge of proper treatment and drug therapy. Insofar as this book mentions any dosage or application, readers may rest assured that the authors, editors, and publishers have made every effort to ensure that such references are in accordance with **the state of knowledge at the time of production of the book.**

Nevertheless, this does not involve, imply, or express any guarantee or responsibility on the part of the publishers in respect to any dosage instructions and forms of applications stated in the book. **Every user is requested to examine carefully** the manufacturers' leaflets accompanying each drug and to check, if necessary in consultation with a physician or specialist, whether the dosage schedules mentioned therein or the contraindications stated by the manufacturers differ from the statements made in the present book. Such examination is particularly important with drugs that are either rarely used or have been newly released on the market. Every dosage schedule or every form of application used is entirely at the user's own risk and responsibility. The authors and publishers request every user to report to the publishers any discrepancies or inaccuracies noticed. If errors in this work are found after publication, errata will be posted at www.thieme.com on the product description page.

Some of the product names, patents, and registered designs referred to in this book are in fact registered trademarks or proprietary names even though specific reference to this fact is not always made in the text. Therefore, the appearance of a name without designation as proprietary is not to be construed as a representation by the publisher that it is in the public domain.

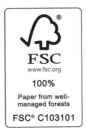

FSC
www.fsc.org
100%
Paper from well-
managed forests
FSC® C103101

This book is dedicated to all of our patients who trust us with their precious vision.

Contents

Foreword

Innumerable presbyopes hoping to minimize spectacle wear employ monovision with contact lenses or leave one eye myopic following LASIK. Likewise, pseudophakic monovision is frequently used as a strategy for presbyopia correction among cataract surgical patients with high satisfaction rates. Recent annual American Society of Cataract and Refractive Surgery (ASCRS) Clinical Surveys suggest that this is a significantly more popular strategy than multifocal IOLs, despite the premium fees associated with the latter. With these facts in mind, it is striking how little print or podium education is devoted to pseudophakic monovision—particularly for cataract and refractive surgeons.

Pseudophakic Monovision: A Clinical Guide is a much-needed comprehensive review of this important, but often omitted, topic. Chief authors Fuxiang Zhang, Alan Sugar, and Graham Barrett are each an authority in this field who combine their vast clinical experience and passion for teaching into a very practical and scientific textbook. In addressing the advantages and drawbacks to this approach, they cover topics ranging from the optics and neurophysiology of monovision to preoperative testing and counseling.

As a topic, pseudophakic monofocal monovision will never have the glamour and sizzle of the next new presbyopia-correcting IOL. Yet, despite how much has been written and discussed about accommodating, multifocal, and extended depth-of-focus (EDOF) IOLs, there is a glaring paucity of clinical studies comparing outcomes and patient satisfaction with these expensive technologies to monofocal monovision. Indeed, ophthalmologists would often select monofocal monovision for their own cataract surgery, according to many informal surveys, in order to avoid compromising quality of vision, particularly at night.

The popularity of pseudophakic monovision is about to change. The FDA recently approved the first adjustable IOL—RxSight's light adjustable IOL. I believe that adjustable IOL technology will disrupt the refractive IOL industry for several reasons. In addition to improving our surgical refractive accuracy, it will allow patients to try out different refractive targets postoperatively in the pseudophakic state, before deciding on their preference prior to the adjustment. Imagine if you could guarantee excellent distance acuity in one eye, and then let the patient test and choose the amount of myopia that works best for their second eye. The pseudophakic patient could even use a soft contact lens trial to experiment with different eye dominance and with different amounts of anisometropia. This would shift the bulk of refractive counseling from pre-op to post-op, and it could be delegated to an optometrist. Most importantly, it would spare patients the confusing and stressful process of deciding what refractive system or outcome they want preoperatively without any ability to try it out. Finally, the refractive IOL adjustment would command a patient premium for postoperative refractive services that are clearly separate from the cataract operation. For all of these reasons, I believe that adjustable IOLs will elevate the popularity of monofocal monovision to new heights.

Lacking industry marketing or sponsored education about monovision, refractive and cataract surgeons will welcome this timely and practical textbook about an essential but relatively neglected topic. It will become a valuable resource as we incorporate new adjustable and EDOF IOL technology into our practices.

David F. Chang, MD

Acknowledgments

This work would not have been possible without my two coauthors. I ran into my teacher and mentor, Alan Sugar, in Cincinnati in 2005 when we were sitting in a classroom for Alcon ReStor certification. We were wondering if the ReStor IOL would be any better than pseudophakic monovision from a patient satisfaction and spectacle independence perspective. Since then, we together started our IOL monovision and refractive cataract surgery research. He has been actively providing me with the protected academic time for all of my research works. I have learned so much from him, not only clinical research skills, but also how to make one's work the highest quality possible. I have had very high respect for Graham Barrett for his leadership in the field of refractive cataract surgery. I truly appreciate his insight and contributions to this book in the last few years. I also want to thank him for his tips and pearls to sharpen my skills in astigmatism management and for sharing his outstanding IOL formulas. I am very fortunate to have these two ophthalmologist giants to work with and to learn from.

I would especially like to thank Warren Hill, David Chang, and Lisa Arbisser for their generous support for allowing me to use their special case reports of IOL monovision contraindications in this book. I am sincerely grateful for their decades-long generous grants of their expertise and advice for my refractive cataract surgery skills. I have learned a lot from them.

Paul Edwards, MD, Chairman of the Department of Ophthalmology at Henry Ford Health System, clearly sees the unique value of IOL monovision in the field of refractive cataract surgery. Without his consistent and strong support, my IOL monovision research projects as well as this book would be impossible. I am very grateful to all of those with whom I have had the pleasure to work at the department of ophthalmology, Henry Ford Health System, in the last 19 years. I would especially like to thank Bithika Kheterpal and Robert Levine, who provided their invaluable feedback from cataract surgeon perspectives before we finalized our last version of the manuscript. Harmonious professional work with my optometry colleagues at Henry Ford Optimeyes has provided me with very strong support for my practice.

My whole staff team at the Downriver Optimeyes Center deserves special thanks for their hard work and outstanding service for our patients and year-round refractive cataract surgery–oriented clinical research. I am especially indebted to the team leader, Lori Cooper, research assistant, Andrea Wood, and our former team members Melissa Collins, Lynn Carter, and Jessica Artico.

The Kellogg Eye Center of the University of Michigan is where I had my second round of ophthalmology residency training from 1994 to 1997. I am using this opportunity to express my gratitude to everyone who taught me and supported me throughout the whole residency training with the Michigan family. I am very thankful for the aspiring guidance, invaluably constructive criticism, and friendly advice during my 3 years there. I am extremely thankful to Paul Lichter, our then chairman, who set the role of model to be a professional, ethical, and caring physician and who was the first one to introduce me to the beauty of the contact lens–induced monovision concept. My deep appreciation goes to Dr. Terry Bergstrom, our then residency program director, who provided me extensive personal support and professional guidance throughout the whole residency. I would especially like to thank Dr. Jonathan Trobe, who taught me how to use a very meticulous and well-organized approach for patient care. I cannot thank Dr. Steve Archer enough for his teaching of optics during my residency. Dr. Archer also graciously reviewed the optical analysis of IOL monovision in Chapter 2 of this book and I am very grateful for this. Special thanks to my fellow residents at the Kellogg Eye Center, Jason Burgett, Stephen Fox, Andrew Hanzlik, Bithika Kheterpal, Michael Kipp, and Amy Neuhoff Robertson, for their inspiration and friendship.

Zhongshan Ophthalmic Center, Sun Yat-san University of Medical Science, Guan Zhou, China, is where I earned my masters degree of medical research in ophthalmic fields from 1985 to 1988. Special thanks go to my mentors, Dr. Eugene Chen, MD, and Professor Dezhen Wu, PhD. I am very thankful for what they taught me, the basic medical and clinical research skills.

The Ophthalmology Department, the School of Medicine, Southeast University, Nanjing, China, is where I received my medical school education and first ophthalmology residency training from 1977 to 1985. I am deeply indebted to the medical school where I learned medicine and became the first MD in my family. My special gratitude goes to the late Dr. Guofan Su and Dr. Qianjin Guan and other teachers and mentors who taught me all the basic ophthalmic knowledge and skills. It is a great pleasure and good fortune to keep a lifelong close relationship with many classmates, with whom I shared our 5-year unforgettable medical-student life.

Thieme is a great publisher to work with. The enthusiasm, trust, and support from the managing team are fantastic, especially from William Lamsback and Elizabeth Palumbo. Without that, it would not have been a seamless process.

Nobody has been more important to me in my professional as well as personal life than the members of my family. Most importantly, I want to sincerely thank my loving and supportive wife, Fenfen, and my two wonderful daughters, Carlen and Carol, and our son-in-law, Kiran, for their understanding and support. Thousands of hours were taken away from weekend and family holiday for my clinical research and in the pursuit of this book, which I deeply appreciate.

Fuxiang Zhang, MD

1 Introduction

Abstract

Presbyopic patients spend money and time to have contact lens monovision or laser vision correction monovision. So why do we cataract surgeons not use intraocular lenses (IOLs) more often to create monovision? For a cataract patient with a desire for spectacle independence after surgery, there are different ways to create monovision. If it were like buying a car, where the prospective buyers can try different models before they make a choice, then IOL monovision might be favored by many more, if not the vast majority of patients, due to the quality of vision from monofocal lenses, low cost, convenience of back up of glasses if needed, and close to negligible downsides.

Monovision as a method of prescribing optical aids was first proposed in 1958 by Richard Westsmith. The first clinical report was from Fonda in 1966. The first known IOL monovision paper was published by Boerner and Thrasher in 1984. IOL monovision is now the most common surgical management of presbyopia for cataract patients. IOL monovision not only can meet patient needs for spectacle independence, but can also build up one's surgical practice and lay a strong foundation for premium IOL refractive cataract surgery. Integrating IOL monovision into premium IOL practice is very helpful or even essential for successful premium refractive cataract surgery. Crossed IOL monovision can be used to rescue one's outcome when the first eye refractive target is missed with accommodative and extended depth of focus IOLs.

Keywords: IOL monovision, pseudophakic monovision, refractive cataract surgery, premium IOL and IOL monovision, clinical outcome of IOL monovision, nighttime driving and monovision, depth perception and monovision, patient satisfaction and monovision, pseudophakic monovision book, IOL monovision book

1.1 Introduction

Monovision is a term used when one eye is intentionally corrected for far and the fellow eye for near. Monovision is a misnomer. It gives the impression of using one eye only or that the two eyes do not work together. The name itself potentially can be a barrier, preventing some patients from considering it as a presbyopia management modality. Blended vision may be a better term. When both eyes work together, monovision provides increased depth of focus but maintains good binocular vision with decreased spectacle independence.

1.2 Why This Book Was Written?

1.2.1 Killing Two Birds with One Stone

People who do not want to wear reading glasses, or cannot wear bifocals, may intentionally use monovision with contact lenses, or may spend thousands of dollars to have laser corneal refractive surgery correction with monovision. Many studies in the literature have demonstrated its validation. Why then do we not use intraocular lenses (IOLs) more often for monovision, one stone killing two birds, when we do cataract surgery? That is the rationale for IOL monovision.

1.2.2 One of the Most Popularly Used Modalities

Increasingly, premium IOLs have become available in the last two decades with the same goal of increasing spectacle independence after cataract surgery, and most of them do well with high patient satisfaction. IOL monovision, however, still stands out with quality of vision, easy adaptation, fewer complications, and less out-of-pocket cost for patients. Modest monovision continues to be an attractive presbyopic solution and, in our opinion, should be considered a "premium" solution. It requires expert surgery, lens selection, and the utilization of toric implants or corneal incisions to reduce astigmatism. From a surgeon's perspective, myopic defocus is one of the two bases of refractive cataract surgery, as expressed in the pyramid scheme in ▶ Fig. 1.1. From a patient perspective, choosing the type of IOL is not like buying a car, where one can try different models and then pick the best. No one will argue that monovision is perfect, with compromises such as fine stereovision, but the truth is that in real life, the negative impact is minimal. (See the section "What Benefits Can IOL Monovision Bring to Your Practice?")

Before we have an ideal accommodating IOL, IOL monovision is still one of the best choices, if not

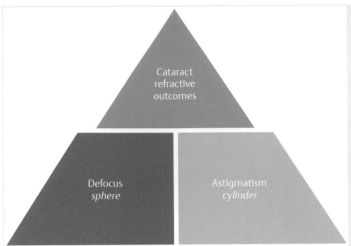

Fig. 1.1 The two main components of refractive cataract surgery. (Courtesy of Alcon Laboratories, Inc., Fort Worth, TX, USA, 2016 AAO Meeting in Chicago, IL.)

the best, in the management of presbyopia among the cataract population. IOL monovision was the number one modality for the management of presbyopia in cataract surgery according to the 2013 ASCRS clinical survey.[1] What is more, the trend of choosing IOL monovision increased between 2013 and 2014.[2]

1.2.3 Residency Education

Most ophthalmology residencies in the United States and the rest of world do not provide formal training for monovision. IOL monovision may not be easy to adopt if one never intentionally has tried it, even though he or she might be a very experienced cataract surgeon. The questions we sometimes get are "How do you know who are good candidates and who are not?" "How much anisometropia should I target?" "What are the contraindications?" From our own learning curve in the practice of IOL monovision, we wished there was a book available which could have provided us some suggestions, pearls, and pitfalls so that we did not have to learn many lessons the hard way.

1.2.4 Making One's Surgical Practice Prosperous

A surgeon who does a large proportion of pseudophakic monovision in cataract surgery for those who desire glasses independence can be expected to have a busy and happy, no-advertisement-needed, prosperous practice, mainly from word of mouth of satisfied patients.

The above are the four main reasons why this book was written. To our knowledge, this is the first book exclusively designated to address IOL monovision.

1.3 A Brief History of Monovision

Monovision as a method of prescribing optical aids was first proposed in 1958 by Richard Westsmith, MD, of San Mateo, California, for presbyopic monocular contact lens wearers.[3] In his paper, he revealed that he had a contact lens of + 1.50 D for his own left eye for reading. He did not need any correction for distance with a vision of 20/20 in each eye. He was unable to tolerate a bifocal for his office work. With monocular contact lens monovision, Westsmith experienced "I have had the contact lens about a month now and I find that I am able to wear it comfortably all day and I have complete clarity of near vision. I am undisturbed by the slight blur in my left eye at distance. With the corneal lens in place, my vision in the left eye is 20/50. However, with both eyes I am able to read J1 at 18 inches. There is no trouble with the ophthalmoscope, retinoscope, or slit lamp."

The first clinical report was from Fonda in 1966 with 13 cases of monovision corrected by spectacles and contact lenses.[4] He also described himself as a monovision user. "I have been wearing a + 3.00 D reading addition before my right eye, and a + 1.50 D reading addition before my left eye for two years. I adjusted immediately to this difference, which does not affect my reading comfort regardless of the circumstances or duration of reading. I can wear a + 2.50 reading addition before one eye and no addition before the other. I have worn a + 2.50 D reading addition before both my dominant left eye and nondominant right eye on different occasions which was accepted equally well. I was conscious of the new correction for less than four hours. I never experienced diplopia, and evidenced fusion by the four-dot test and the Wirt stereo-quantitative test."

The first known pseudophakic monovision paper was published by Boerner and Thrasher in 1984.[5] In that study, among the 100 IOL monovision patients, the need to have bifocals after the surgery decreased 50%. And IOL monovision is now the most common surgical management of presbyopia for cataract patients.[1,2]

For the last half century, monovision has been increasingly used for presbyopia management with an impressive success rate. There are different ways to provide monovision: spectacles, contact lenses, refractive lasers, intraocular implants, etc. This book concentrates on the discussion of IOL monovision, or pseudophakic monovision, but at the same time, other methods will be briefly discussed, since most of the monovision studies in the literature were with contact lens and laser vision correction. IOL monovision is barely discussed in the literature considering how widely it is used in our profession.

1.4 What Benefits Can Pseudophakic Monovision Bring to Your Practice?

1.4.1 To Meet Patients' Needs

We used to be satisfied with regular telegraphy and then telephones, but now we are happier with smart phones and the internet. Science and technology will continue to advance. Cataract surgery was simply a vision rehabilitation procedure a few decades ago, but it is not so any more. Just from a spectacle independence point of view, our clinical survey (all the 441 cataract patients' 697 eyes in 2016) noted that 44% of our cataract patients would like to have some level of freedom from glasses and nearly one-fourth would like to have complete glasses independence. If financial factors were not considered, these percentages would be expected to be much higher.

1.4.2 To Build Up Practice

About 10 years ago, one of my junior staff members called me (F. Z.) at home. He was wondering why his practice was not as busy since he had joined our health system a few years earlier and he wanted me to give him advice in terms of what

made my practice very busy while we were in the same geographic area. My answer was "Do your best to satisfy your patients and do IOL monovision." Our own comparative prospective studies proved slightly better overall performance and satisfaction in IOL monovision than multifocal IOL patients.[6,7] When compared with premium IOLs, IOL monovision has a few obvious advantages:

1. High patient satisfaction. As mentioned below, our 10-year IOL monovision review with a de-identified survey noted 97% satisfaction. Anecdotal experience of IOL monovision success from Bill Maloney, one of the IOL monovision pioneers, was 99%.[8]
2. Use of monofocal IOLs with high vision quality. Many fewer complaints and very low IOL explantation rate. Downside in real life is negligible.
3. Back up glasses are very handy when the need arises to have full binocular vision.
4. Less or no direct patient cost.

These advantages are significant and word of mouth is the most powerful advertisement in the community. If one's surgical complications are also very low, then one can expect a busy practice.

Overall, IOL monovision clinical outcomes can be excellent if we master all the key steps. We did a de-identified survey of all of our IOL monovision patients over 10 years. All 5,660 charts of consecutive cataract surgical cases performed by F. Z. from January 2005 to December 2014 were reviewed (followed up to August 2015). Among 359 qualified cases, 194 were enrolled, 30 had died, 48 declined participation, and the remaining 87 could not be contacted with at least three phone calls. Among the 48 who declined participation, the vast majority did not have regular postoperative follow-up.

The mean age was 72.5 years. The subjects were 135 females (69.6%) and 59 males (30.4%). Mean follow-up was nearly 3 years (35 months). Mean distance vision without correction for the distance eye was 20/24.7 and mean near vision without correction for the near eye was 20/28.1. Mean anisometropia was 1.30 D.

To ensure accountability and reliability, it was clearly described in the introduction of the survey letter to each patient that the surgeon is not going to have access to the survey and thus to kindly provide honest opinion. All the original data of the survey were handled by a research assistant, and the statistics were then performed by an independent statistician. The four brief outcomes of the survey are shown as follows (▶ Fig. 1.2, ▶ Fig. 1.3, ▶ Fig. 1.4, ▶ Fig. 1.5).

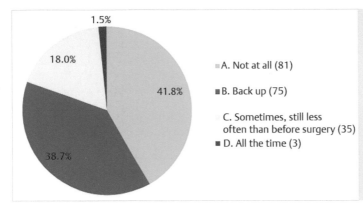

Fig. 1.2 Spectacle independence, glasses use. (The number in parentheses is the patient number.)

1.5%

18.0%

41.8%

38.7%

- A. Not at all (81)
- B. Back up (75)
- C. Sometimes, still less often than before surgery (35)
- D. All the time (3)

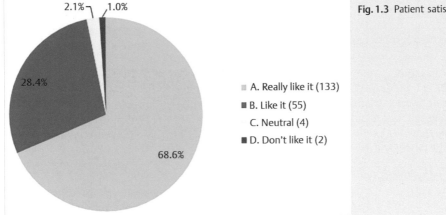

Fig. 1.3 Patient satisfaction.

2.1% 1.0%

28.4%

68.6%

- A. Really like it (133)
- B. Like it (55)
- C. Neutral (4)
- D. Don't like it (2)

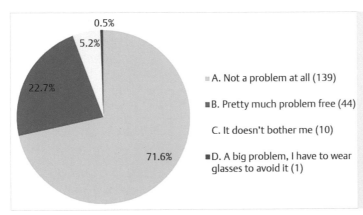

Fig. 1.4 Depth perception problems without glasses or contact lenses.

0.5%

5.2%

22.7%

71.6%

- A. Not a problem at all (139)
- B. Pretty much problem free (44)
- C. It doesn't bother me (10)
- D. A big problem, I have to wear glasses to avoid it (1)

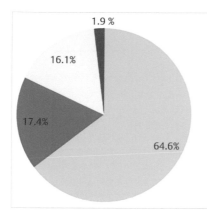

Fig. 1.5 Nighttime driving problems without glasses or contact lenses.

- A. No need to wear glasses and I have no problem (104)
- B. Need glasses only if heavy traffic or bad weather (28)
- C. Need glasses for all nighttime driving (26)
- D. Don't drive at nighttime due to vision problems (3)

1.9 %
16.1%
17.4%
64.6%

1.4.3 To Lay a Solid Foundation for Refractive Cataract Surgery

IOL monovision works well, but it is not perfect. It is not the summit of technology. Surgeons have to keep an open mind and keep trying new technology rather than become stale, otherwise they will fall behind. But we should not stick to new things if they are not really working as well as claimed, or if they are not as good as the old ones. In other words, we have to follow the rules of evidence-based practice.

Once one intentionally plans to use IOL monovision, one will have to be fully engaged to improve biometry accuracy, skills in astigmatism correction with toric IOLs or limbal relaxing incisions, and overall surgical skills and outcomes, otherwise one cannot expect good monovision results. These are essentially the same components as for premium IOL practice with differences in preoperative patient selection and consultation.

Why do we refer to IOL monovision as the foundation for refractive cataract surgery? It is because

1. This can be one's starting point, because IOL monovision is more forgiving than premium IOL use, especially for the nondominant eye.
2. Monovision costs less out of pocket, so expectations may not be too high to meet.
3. If one does not have a track record of accurate biometry and does not feel comfortable with astigmatism correction, the chance of successful premium IOL refractive surgery is low. Starting premium IOL surgery unprepared, with subsequent case failures, will have a high chance of leading one to abandon these new methods. Hitting the refractive target is one of the keys for IOL monovision success. It involves all the steps. For example, if everything has

been optimized, but the IOL formula is still an outdated version, then the outcome may still not be as good as expected. That is the concept of mean absolute error.[9]

4. Integrating IOL monovision into premium IOL practice is very helpful or even essential for successful premium refractive cataract surgery. (See the section "Premium IOLs and IOL Monovision" in Chapter 4.) Crossed IOL monovision can be used to rescue one's outcome when the first eye refractive target is missed in accommodative and extended depth of focus IOLs.

References

[1] ASCRS Clinical Survey 2013. EyeWorld Vol. 18, Number 11. November 20, 2013
[2] Lindstrom RL. Pursuit of ideal presbyopia-correcting IOL continues. Ocular Surgery News October 10, 2015:4–5
[3] Westsmith RA. Uses of a monocular contact lens. Am J Ophthalmol. 1958; 46(1, Pt 1):78–81
[4] Fonda G. Presbyopia corrected with single vision spectacles or corneal lenses in preference to bifocal corneal lenses. Trans Ophthalmol Soc Aust. 1966; 25:78–80
[5] Boerner CF, Thrasher BH. Results of monovision correction in bilateral pseudophakes. J Am Intraocul Implant Soc. 1984; 10(1):49–50
[6] Zhang F, Sugar A, Jacobsen G, Collins M. Visual function and patient satisfaction: comparison between bilateral diffractive multifocal intraocular lenses and monovision pseudophakia. J Cataract Refract Surg. 2011; 37(3):446–453
[7] Zhang F, Sugar A, Jacobsen G, Collins M. Visual function and spectacle independence after cataract surgery: bilateral diffractive multifocal intraocular lenses versus monovision pseudophakia. J Cataract Refract Surg. 2011; 37(5):853–858
[8] Maloney WF. Monovision with monofocal IOLs. In: Chang DF, ed. Mastering Refractive IOLs: The Art and Science. Thorofare, NJ: Slack Incorporated; 2008:448–449
[9] Hill WE. Hitting emmetropia. In: Chang DF, ed. Mastering Refractive IOLs: The Art and Science. Thorofare, NJ: Slack Incorporated; 2008:533–534

2 Optics and Neurophysiology of Pseudophakic Monovision

Abstract

By choosing appropriate intraocular lens (IOL) power differences between the two eyes, we can create IOL monovision in such a way that the depth of focus is increased within the physiological range with minimal compromise. Mini and modest monovision are likely more physiological situations where binocular summation rather than monocular blur suppression plays the main role. Optically, it is also demonstrable that the not-sharply-focused-zone is shorter in −1.50 D monovision than −2.50 D monovision. The hole-in-card sighting dominance test likely reflects more the monocular situation, while the plus lens sensory test reflects more binocular perception and balance.

Keywords: IOL monovision, pseudophakic monovision, mini monovision, modest monovision, full or traditional monovision, depth perception, not-sharply-focus-zone, hole-in-card, plus-lens test, dominant eye test

The main purpose of designing IOL monovision is to increase depth of focus to eliminate or decrease spectacle dependence by choosing different IOL powers in the two eyes. A successful IOL monovision patient should be able to see at all distances, spanning from the far focal point of the far eye when the eye is not accommodating to the near focal point of the near eye when the eye is accommodating, although in optical theory there may be a zone where there is no sharp focus.

If a patient's eyes are both phakic and emmetropic at the age of 60, with an average accommodative amplitude of 1.00 D at that age, that patient will be able to see well from 20 feet away to infinity when the eyes are not accommodating (lights coming from 20 feet and farther away are considered as zero vergence power, or parallel to the optic axis ray),[1] but for near, he or she will be able to focus only up to 1 m in front of him or her, not any closer without an optical addition (▶ Fig. 2.1).

2.1 Optics of Increased Depth of Focus

The first symptoms of presbyopia—eyestrain, difficulty seeing in dim light, and problems focusing on fine print—are usually noticed between the ages of 40 and 45. The ability to focus on near objects declines throughout life, from an accommodative amplitude of about 20 D (ability to focus at 5 cm) in a child, to about 10 D at age 25 (10 cm), and levels off at 0.50 to 1.00 D at age 60 (ability to focus down to 1–2 m only).

2.1.1 Equation 1

Near focal point of each eye $(N) = 100/1$ D
$$= 100 \text{ cm}$$
$$= 1 \text{ m}$$

If the patient's status is now post cataract surgery with plano in each eye with 20/20 distance vision in each eye, assuming natural nonaccommodating pseudophakic accommodation power of 1.00 D for each eye, he or she will still see well 20 feet away, but at near he or she will only be able to focus up to about 1 m, not any closer with the same formula and calculation as above (▶ Fig. 2.2).

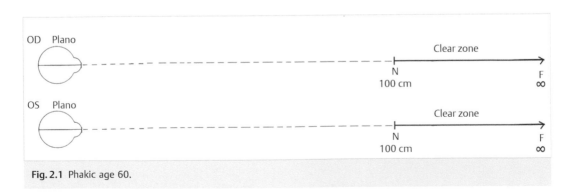

Fig. 2.1 Phakic age 60.

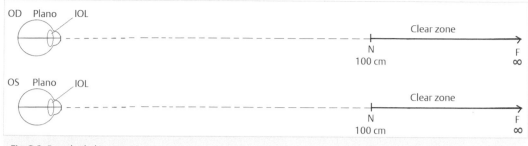

Fig. 2.2 Pseudophakic age 60.

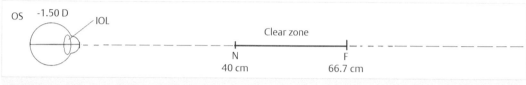

Fig. 2.3 OS –1.50 pseudophakic.

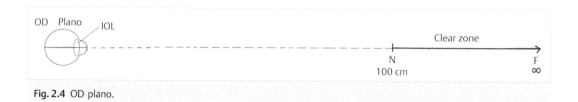

Fig. 2.4 OD plano.

2.1.2 Anisometropia –1.50 D Monovision

If we keep the patient's OD the same, at plano, but give the OS more myopic defocus, say adding extra power to the IOL to give the patient –1.50 D monovision (for the sake of discussion simplicity, we do give two different powers at IOL plane and at glasses plane, although we all know that when we add + 1.00 D to the IOL typically we will get roughly about 2/3 D at the glasses level), then the patient's OS will have a focusing power of 2.50 D (extra 1.50 D + 1.00 D from assumed pseudophakic accommodation = 2.50 D) with a new near focal point of 40 cm in front of him/her.

2.1.3 Equation 2

Near focal point of OS (*N*) = 100/2.5 D
= 40 cm
= About 16 inches

2.1.4 Equation 3

Far focal point of OS (*F*) = 100/1.5 D
= 66.7 cm
= About 26 inches

Clear zone of OS is between 40 and 66.7 cm (▶ Fig. 2.3).

The patient's OD should be able to see clearly from infinity to up to 100 cm with this eye due to assumed pseudophakic accommodation of 1.00 D.

2.1.5 Equation 4

Near focal point of OD (*N*) = 100/1 D
= 100 cm
= About 39 inches

2.1.6 Equation 5

Far focal point of OD (*F*) = infinity

Clear zone of OD is 100 cm to infinity (▶ Fig. 2.4).

Thus, the patient should be able to see well in the range from infinity to 40 cm in front of him or her when both eyes are working together. That is what we mean when we say that IOL monovision increases the depth of focus (▶ Fig. 2.5).

Optically, the left eye's far focal point is not at infinity any more. It is at 66.7 cm in front of the patient. Any farther away, the OS alone is not able to see sharply without myopic correction for the left eye. That is the compromise of monovision. This is actually the most common "negative" comment from IOL monovision patients if it is not clearly explained to them prior to the surgery. However, the reality of IOL monovision in this scenario is that they see well for both far and near and in between without much noticeable downside in daily life since we live our lives with both eyes open, although optically in theory there is still a zone that is not in sharp focus. This concept is helpful when we discuss the pros and cons of modest versus high anisometropia.

Not-Sharply-Focused-Zone

What happens if the object is located at 50 cm in front of the patient? His or her OD alone is not going to focus well since the refraction is plano, although the assumed pseudophakic accommodation of 1.00 D will enable the right eye to see everything clearly from infinity to up to 100 cm away to the eye. The object located at 50 cm is within the clear zone of OS (40–66.7 cm) (▶ Fig. 2.6).

What happens if the object is located at 75 cm in front of the patient? It is located within the not-sharply-focused-zone (NSFZ).

The NSFZ is defined as the distance between the near focal point of the distance eye and the far focal point of the near eye in monovision.

The length of the NSFZ is 33.3 cm between 100 and 66.7 cm when we create –1.50 D IOL monovision (▶ Fig. 2.7).

Optically, within the "NSFZ," neither the OD nor the OS will have perfectly sharp focus. This is the compromise of monovision when the anisometropia level gets high. It may have some negative impact in full monovision, but it is close to negligible at mini and modest monovision.

2.1.7 Anisometropia –2.50 D Monovision

Now, what if the anisometropic level is –2.50 D, instead of –1.50 D for the OS? Let us assume the right eye is still plano with pseudophakic accommodation amplitude of 1.00 D. The total focusing power for OS will be 2.50 + 1.00 = 3.50 D.

2.1.8 Equation 6

Near focal point of OS (N) = 100/3.5 D
$$= 28.6 \text{ cm}$$
$$= \text{About 11 inches}$$

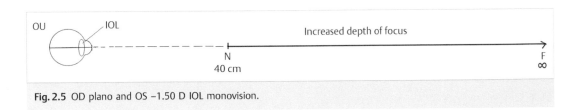

Fig. 2.5 OD plano and OS –1.50 D IOL monovision.

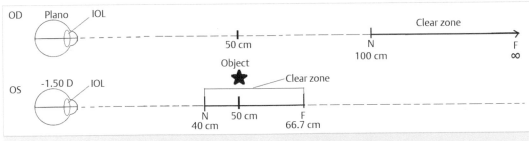

Fig. 2.6 The object is located at 50 cm in front of the eye within the clear zone of OS.

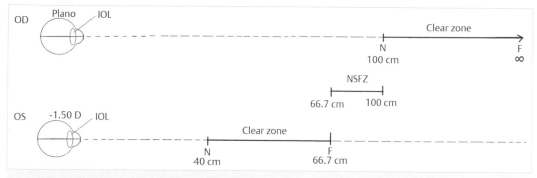

Fig. 2.7 Concept of NSFZ in –1.50 D IOL monovision.

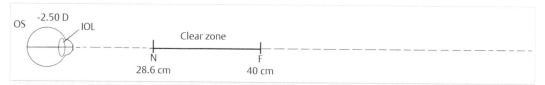

Fig. 2.8 OS with –2.50 D pseudophakic, near point and far point without correction.

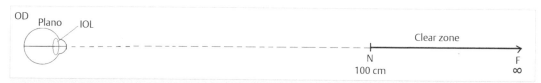

Fig. 2.9 OD plano pseudophakic.

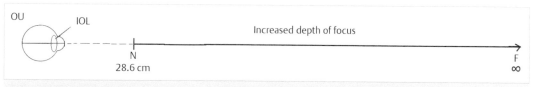

Fig. 2.10 OD plano and OS –2.50 D IOL monovision.

2.1.9 Equation 7

Far focal point of OS (F) = 100/2.5 D

$\qquad$ = 40 cm

$\qquad$ = About 15.6 inches

The clear focusable zone of OS is between 28.6 and 40 cm (▶ Fig. 2.8).

Patient's OD should be able to see clearly from infinity to up to 100 cm with the eye due to assumed pseudophakic accommodation of 1.00 D.

2.1.10 Equation 8

Near focal point of OD (N) = 100/1 D

$\qquad$ = 100 cm

$\qquad$ = About 39 inches

2.1.11 Equation 5

Far focal point of OD (F) = infinity

The clear focusable zone of OD is 100 cm to infinity (▶ Fig. 2.9).

Therefore, the depth of focus is from infinity to 28.6 cm in front of him/her when both eyes are working together if OS is –2.50 D monovision (▶ Fig. 2.10).

Optically, the left eye's far focal point is not at infinity any more. It is at 40 cm in front of the patient. Anything farther away, the OS alone is not able to see sharply without myopic correction of the left eye. That is again the compromise of monovision.

Not-Sharply-Focused-Zone with −2.50D Monovision

Let us take a look again when the object is located at 50 cm in front of him. His OD alone is not going to focus well on the object since the refraction is plano, although the assumed pseudophakic accommodation of 1.00 D will enable the right eye to see everything clearly from infinity to up to 100 cm away with the eye. The object located at 50 cm is *not* within the clear zone of OS anymore since the clear zone of OS is now between 28.6 and 40 cm. When the IOL monovision is −1.50 D, the clear zone for the OS is from 40 to 66.7 cm.

The object located at 75 cm in front of the patient is still located within the NSFZ with −2.50 D IOL monovision.

The length of the NSFZ now is 60 cm, between 100 and 40 cm when −2.50 D IOL monovision is created (▶ Fig. 2.11).

The length of the NSFZ becomes longer at −2.50 D anisometropia than at −1.50 D anisometropia monovision. When we give −1.50 D to OS as IOL monovision, the length of the NSFZ is 33.3 cm, between 100 and 66.7 cm. Thus, the difference in length of the NSFZ between −1.50 D IOL monovision and −2.50 D IOL monovision is close to doubled (60 vs. 33.3 cm).

The concept of the NSFZ is related to the nature of a rigid lens versus the natural human lens as well as age.

IOL versus Natural Lens

Let us take a look at an example of 20/20 plano OD and 20/20 OS with −1.50 D monovision in a 50-year-old man, but with natural *phakic* monovision, instead of *pseudophakic* monovision. His OD clear zone is from infinity to 50 cm, assuming accommodation amplitude of 2.00 D for a 50-year-old.

2.1.12 Equation 9

Near focal point of OD $(N) = 100/2$ D
$$= 50 \, \text{cm}$$

2.1.13 Equation 5

Far focal point of OD (F) = infinity (▶ Fig. 2.12)

His OS clear zone is from 66.7 cm when the OS is not accommodating to 28.6 cm when the OS is accommodating. There is no NSFZ in this scenario.

2.1.14 Equation 10

Near focal point of OS $(N) = 100/(1.5 + 2)$ D
$$= 28.6 \, \text{cm}$$

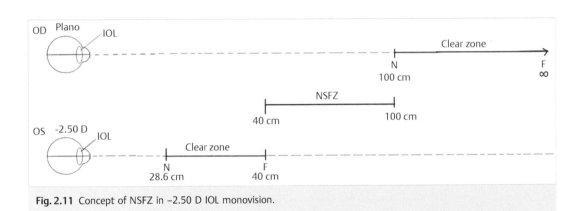

Fig. 2.11 Concept of NSFZ in −2.50 D IOL monovision.

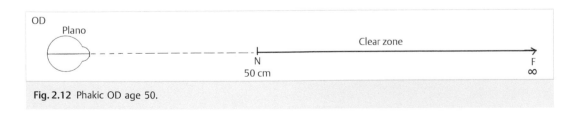

Fig. 2.12 Phakic OD age 50.

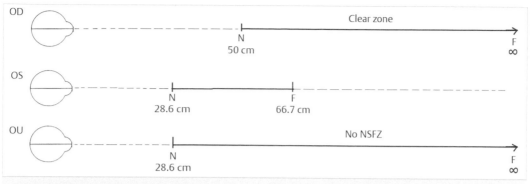

Fig. 2.13 Phakic monovision age 50.

2.1.15 Equation 11

Far focal point of OS (F) = 100/1.5 D

= 66.7 cm (▶ Fig. 2.13)

If his monovision were with IOLs rather than natural accommodating lenses, the number "2" in the above denominators for OD as well as OS would be "1" since the IOL does not have the ability to change power, assuming younger pseudophakic patients also have average pseudophakic accommodation of 1.00 D. The nature of the natural lens with the ability to increase its curvature when the eye is accommodating makes the near focal point closer.

Age

Because of the age (50 years), he has 2.00 D accommodative amplitude versus 1.00 D at age 60.

Optically, within the "NSFZ," neither the OD nor the OS will have perfectly sharp focus. The length of the NSFZ gets longer as the anisometropic level increases. This again is the compromise of IOL monovision. This may also be one of the contributing factors to why full monovision at the –2.50 D level may require greater compromise than modest monovision at the –1.25 D to –1.50 D level. For example, full monovision patients may need to sit closer to read the computer clearly when they do not wear any glasses. The computer might be located in the NSFZ if they do not move closer. For further discussions see the section "How Much Anisometropia Works Best?" in Chapter 4.

2.2 Why High Anisometropia May Require Greater Compromise

Binocular vision is when creatures having two eyes use them together. Humans have a maximum

horizontal field of view of approximately 190 degrees with two eyes, in approximately 120 degrees of which a binocular field of view is possible, flanked by two uniocular fields (seen by only one eye) of approximately 40 degrees.[2] This can give stereopsis in which binocular disparity provided by the two eyes' different positions in the head gives precise depth perception, but Panum's fusional area only has a small volume of visual space around where the eyes are fixating.

Theoretically, when there are two fields of view, there is a potential for confusion between the left and right eye's images of the same object, if the disparity is too great. This can be dealt with in three ways: one image can be suppressed, so that only one image is seen, or the two images can be fused; if fusion and/or suppression do not happen, two images of a single object are seen, and diplopia occurs. Fortunately, in the vast majority of IOL monovision patients, if the anisometropia level is reasonable, there is no diplopia. In mini-monovision (–.50 – –0.75D) and modest monovision, when the disparity is small, bilateral summation (binocular summation is defined as the superiority of visual function for binocular over monocular viewing)[3] is likely dominant. As the anisometropia level increases, automatic suppression by the brain may become necessary. When that happens, it may be mainly in a small central area to avoid confusion, while the periphery is unsuppressed to provide binocular vision.[4] This has been the traditional explanation. This kind of suppression probably becomes necessary when the anisometropic level becomes large enough, as in full monovision at 1.75 to 2.50 D. What is more, if we are aiming for –2.50 D for the near eye refractive target, it is not rare to have the final refractive outcome 0.50 D off from our goal. Usually, 3.00 D anisometropia should be avoided for most patients in IOL monovision practice. With modest monovision at or lower than 1.50 D, binocular summation is likely more active than unilateral suppression. Decreasing the aniso-metropia level decreases the NSFZ (see the section "Optics of Increased Depth of Focus" earlier in this chapter).

Consider that for every 0.25 D difference in refraction between the two eyes, there is a 0.5% difference in image size (aniseikonia). If the anisometropia is 2.50 D, then the image size difference will be 5%, which is usually the accepted limit for binocular vision.[5] Generally speaking, −1.25 D to −1.50 D defocus is a preferred arrangement.[6,7,8,9,10,11,12] More than 1.50 D can have a more significant impact on stereovision and contrast sensitivity. See more discussions in the section "How Much Anisometropia Works Best?" in Chapter 4.

2.3 Why Is a Sighting Dominance Test Usually Used for Clinical Decision-Making?

Preoperative clinically dominant eye tests for monovision can be divided into two basic groups. One is a sighting dominance test and one is a sensory dominance test. The subject is forced to choose one eye over the fellow eye in the sighting dominance test while the subject is asked about his or her balance and perceptual preference in the sensory dominance test. The sighting dominance test contains stereo-objects with a disparity beyond Panum's area, while sensory dominance, also referred to as ocular prevalence, is determined using stereo-targets imaged within Panum's area.[13] Between the two types of tests, there is no simple conclusion in terms of correlation. That means the sighting dominant eye is not always the sensory dominant eye.[7,13,14,15,16,17,18]

The hole-in-card test (see the section "Preoperative Tests for Pseudophakic Monovision" in Chapter 4) was found to be the most commonly used sighting dominance test and the plus lens test the most commonly used sensory dominance test.[16] The sighting dominance test seems to be more related to the monocular condition. Our anecdotal experience seems to suggest that usually when one eye is habitually dominant for distance, the chance of successful IOL monovision is very good if we keep it as the distance eye after the cataract surgery.

A study[19] using fMRI (functional magnetic resonance imaging) has demonstrated significantly higher cortical activation in response to stimulation of the dominant eye, defined by sighting, than to stimulation of the nondominant eye. In a separate study,[20] fMRI showed significantly higher cortical activation in response to the dominant eye than the nondominant eye when defined by visual acuity. In clinical settings, sighting dominance is typically correlated with vision, meaning the distance dominant eye is typically the better vision eye, but that is not always the case. Studies[21] of normal cats with monocular vision deprivation for the first 2 to 3 months of life found out that most cells of the striate cortex receive input from both eyes, but the input from the dominant eye produces a greater response to a given stimulus than the input from the nondominant eye.

The sensory dominance test is technically a binocular test, in which the subject is tested for perception and balance and overall feeling. Because of the equal decussation of optic tract anatomy, each hemisphere in the brain receives equal ocular information from both the right and the left. A well-designed study done by Ooi and He[18] suggested that the interocular imbalance caused by sensory dominance is largely attributable to processing by the binocular channel, not the monocular channel, since monocular input of either contrast or brightness did not correlate to sensory dominance.

References

[1] Jose RT. Understanding Low Vision. New York, NY: American Foundation for the Blind; 1983:187–210
[2] Henson DB. Visual Fields. Oxford: Oxford University Press; 1993
[3] Pineles SL, Velez FG, Isenberg SJ, et al. Functional burden of strabismus: decreased binocular summation and binocular inhibition. JAMA Ophthalmol. 2013; 131(11):1413–1419
[4] Key JE, Rigel LE. Monovision Guidelines for Success. Continuing Education for Optometrists & Opticians. Elkins Park, PA: Pennsylvania College of Optometry; 1994 [sponsored by Johnson & Johnson Vision Products, Inc.]
[5] Duke-Elder S, Abrams D. System of Ophthalmology. Vol. 5. Anisometropia. St. Louis, MO: C.V. Mosby Co.; 1970
[6] Pollard ZF, Greenberg MF, Bordenca M, Elliott J, Hsu V. Strabismus precipitated by monovision. Am J Ophthalmol. 2011; 152(3):479–482.e1
[7] Evans BJ. Monovision: a review. Ophthalmic Physiol Opt. 2007; 27(5):417–439
[8] Zhang F, Sugar A, Arbisser L, Jacobsen G, Artico J. Crossed versus conventional pseudophakic monovision: Patient satisfaction, visual function, and spectacle independence. J Cataract Refract Surg. 2015; 41(9):1845–1854
[9] Hayashi K, Yoshida M, Manabe S, Hayashi H. Optimal amount of anisometropia for pseudophakic monovision. J Refract Surg. 2011; 27(5):332–338
[10] Hayashi K, Ogawa S, Manabe S, Yoshimura K. Binocular visual function of modified pseudophakic monovision. Am J Ophthalmol. 2015; 159(2):232–240
[11] Pardhan S, Gilchrist J. The effect of monocular defocus on binocular contrast sensitivity. Ophthalmic Physiol Opt. 1990; 10(1):33–36

[12] Loshin DS, Loshin MS, Comer G. Binocular summation with monovision contact lens correction for presbyopia. Int Contact Lens Clin. 1982; 9:161–165

[13] Kommerell G, Schmitt C, Kromeier M, Bach M. Ocular prevalence versus ocular dominance. Vision Res. 2003; 43(12): 1397–1403

[14] Schor C, Carson M, Peterson G, Suzuki J, Erickson P. Effects of interocular blur suppression ability on monovision task performance. J Am Optom Assoc. 1989; 60(3):188–192

[15] Pointer JS. The absence of lateral congruency between sighting dominance and the eye with better visual acuity. Ophthalmic Physiol Opt. 2007; 27(1):106–110

[16] Seijas O, Gómez de Liaño P, Gómez de Liaño R, Roberts CJ, Piedrahita E, Diaz E. Ocular dominance diagnosis and its influence in monovision. Am J Ophthalmol. 2007; 144(2):209–216

[17] Handa T, Mukuno K, Uozato H, Niida T, Shoji N, Shimizu K. Effects of dominant and nondominant eyes in binocular rivalry. Optom Vis Sci. 2004; 81(5):377–383

[18] Ooi TL, He ZJ. Sensory eye dominance. Optometry. 2001; 72(3): 168–178

[19] Rombouts SA, Barkhof F, Sprenger M, Valk J, Scheltens P. The functional basis of ocular dominance: functional MRI (fMRI) findings. Neurosci Lett. 1996; 221(1):1–4

[20] Mendola JD, Conner IP. Eye dominance predicts fMRI signals in human retinotopic cortex. Neurosci Lett. 2007; 414(1): 30–34

[21] Pearlman AL. The central visual pathways. In: Moses RA, Hart WM, eds. Adler's Physiology of the Eye: Clinical Applications. St Louis, MO: CV Mosby; 1987:583–618

3 Non-Pseudophakic Monovision

Abstract

For patients with natural monovision, it is important to rule out amblyopia and monofixation syndrome; otherwise, they can be excellent candidates for intraocular lens monovision. Both contact lens–induced monovision and laser vision correction–induced monovision work very well in terms of patient satisfaction and spectacle independence. Because of frame/prism-induced downsides, spectacle-induced monovision is not commonly used. Because of the concern for its durability, conductive keratoplasty is no longer a popular modality to create monovision.

Keywords: natural monovision, spectacle-induced monovision, contact lens monovision, laser vision monovision, conductive keratoplasty monovision

3.1 Natural Monovision

Sometimes, we may see patients who present with natural anisometropia, one eye good for far and one eye good for near with no contact lenses or any previous history of refractive surgery. If the patient is also of presbyopic age and has good vision in both eyes, one for distance and one for near without glasses, contact lenses, or amblyopia, we may consider this to be "natural monovision."

Natural monovision does not necessarily mean these patients were born with that same level of anisometropia. As we know, it is very easy for a young child with anisometropia to develop amblyopia if anisometropia is great enough.

A study of 411 children by Weakley noted spherical myopic anisometropia of > 2.00 D or spherical hyperopic anisometropia of > 1.00 D resulted in a statistically significant increase in amblyopia and decrease in bifixation when compared to nonanisometropic patients.[1] It was also noted that if there is anisometropia of > 1.50 D of hyperopia and > 3.00 D of myopia, it will be more likely to make a young child amblyopic.[2] In terms of monofixation syndrome, anisometropia > 1.50 D will put a child at a 50% risk of becoming a monofixator; > 2.00 D will increase the risk to almost 100%.[2]

Thus, those patients presenting as "natural monovision" in the office at cataract age with good foveal fusion and stereopsis without monofixation syndrome might not necessarily have been born with that same level of anisometropia. These patients are lucky from a glasses independence point of view for most of their lifespan. Evans[3] also noted that those patients could do well without any glasses or contact lenses for both far and near. The dominant eye typically has good distance vision but the near vision eye may need some myopic lens correction if good distance vision is required. As they age, their crystalline lenses will change, which may cause their refractive status to change. The stereovision for these natural monovision individuals can be expected to be perfect or nearly perfect with 40 seconds of arc at near without glasses or contact lenses.

The clinical importance for these patients is twofold: the clinician should be cautious to make sure that no monofixation and amblyopia exists; and these may be the best candidates for intraocular lens (IOL) monovision when they need cataract surgery should they want to maintain a high level of spectacle independence.

As an example, I (F. Z.) have always had good vision. My uncorrected distance vision was 20/20 with my right eye and better than 20/15 (1.33 in decimal) with my left eye without glasses on my college entrance physical examination. My right eye probably had mild myopia but I never had a refraction before I became an ophthalmologist since I did not have any eye problem. In my 40 s, I noticed more myopic change in my right eye, while my left eye, the dominant eye, remained plano until my mid-50 s. Up to my mid-50 s, my right eye was –1.50 D sphere and my left eye was plano, and I was doing well with natural monovision without any readers until my mid-50 s. I did not have to wear reading glasses until age 57 when I noticed mild difficulty with small print and my refraction at that time was: right eye –1.00 D and left eye + 0.50 D, which I believe was due to my early cataract formation. My unaided Titmus stereovision was 40 seconds of arc at age 57. My unaided Worth Four-Dot test has always been normal at near as well at 20 feet. A cover and uncover test showed 4 PD exophoria at distance in primary gaze. I have worn single vision + 1.50 D readers for most of my regular size print reading since age 57. Over-the-counter + 1.50 D works just fine. I did wear a pair of single vision glasses for distance during my residency training at the Kellogg Eye Center of the University of Michigan in Ann Arbor in my late 30 s, mainly to bring the right eye to plano. I do have distance glasses when I am driving at night but I do not have to use them. For most nighttime driving, I do not use them, although I typically use them in bad weather conditions. I have never worn bifocals, since most of the time I do not need help from glasses for distance activities.

3.2 Contact Lens Monovision

Contact lens monovision was practiced much earlier than IOL monovision, and many literature citations in this book are from contact lens monovision. Monovision was first proposed by Richard Westmith, MD, of California in 1958 when he fit a +1.50 D contact lens for his own left eye for reading, while his right was the dominant eye for distance without a contact lens. His unaided distance vision was 20/20 in each eye.[4] The first reported clinical study of contact lens monovision was by Fonda[5] in 1966, who also used different powers of add in his bifocals.

The advantages of contact lenses over spectacles are improved cosmetics, decreased peripheral distortion, less aniseikonia, and increased field of view. In spite of the compromise of slightly decreased stereovision, some studies[6,7] suggested that monovision contact lens correction was the most successful and most popular presbyopic management modality when compared with other presbyopic contact lens management, such as bifocal contact lenses. Evans[3] reviewed more than 100 publications to evaluate the literature on the use of monovision for correction of presbyopia. The overall success rate with contact lenses was 59 to 67%. This is obviously lower than the rate from corneal laser vision correction monovision of 72 to 97.6%.[8,9,10] Contact lens wear itself is a dynamic process and contact lens handling can certainly have an impact on the success rate. Contact lens monovision has a higher rate of failure if we include the factor of contact lens intolerance. A literature review by Jain et al[10] noted that the success rate increased from 69 to 81% if the contact lens intolerance factor was excluded. The variable success rates reported might be due to differing criteria used to define success and variations in study duration, ambiguous definitions of the base population, and lack of criteria for minimum contact lens–wearing times.

Contact lens–induced monovision was also demonstrated to be successful for management of symptomatic diplopia.[11,12,13] It is one of the options to alleviate diplopia for patients who failed conventional prism correction. See details in the section "Monovision to Correct Diplopia" in Chapter 5.

3.3 Spectacle Monovision

Spectacle monovision with different powers for both distance correction and the reading add was employed in the 1960s to correct aphakia and it was demonstrated to be successful.[5,14] Because of vertex distance, spectacle monovision creates more aniseikonia and prismatic effect than contact lens monovision, refractive cornea surgery, and IOL monovision. If the anisometropia is 2.75 D, the aniseikonia created with a contact lens would be 0.5%, while with spectacles it would be about 6%.[15] Another reason why spectacle monovision is not popular is that the main reason for having monovision is to decrease or eliminate dependence on glasses, so wearing glasses for monovision does not have much value.

The earliest literature about spectacle monovision was in 1966 by Gerald Fonda, MD, of New Jersey.[5] He reported 13 cases of monovision correction with spectacles and contact lenses. Eleven out of the 13 were successful. Dr. Fonda noted "By the use of corneal lenses the difference between corrections readily acceptable is much greater, because there is less difference in the retinal image size. There is a 22% difference in image size when the average monocular aphakia is corrected with a spectacle lens, and an 8% difference when corrected with a corneal lens." Dr. Fonda himself had "unequal reading additions of +3.00 D right eye and +1.50 D left eye." Of note, Dr. Fonda was also a pioneer for low vision work. I (F. Z.) am very grateful for his influence on my career growth. He sent his book *Management of Low Vision* and one Visolett magnifier to me in December 1986 when I was still in China pursuing my master's degree in postdoctoral research training. That book taught me much of my basic optical knowledge. I was fortunate to meet him in New Jersey in the fall of 1989. Dr. Gerald Fonda passed away at age 86 on January 4, 1996. His contributions to low vision and to monovision will last forever.

Monovision glasses with an anisometropic level of 2.50 or 3.00 D were also purposely used to correct longstanding acquired small-angle (<10 PD) secondary diplopia.[11] Twenty patients age 45 and older were studied with monovision correction to further dampen symptomatic diplopia. Their dominant eye was corrected for distance and nondominant eye for near with either a +2.50 D or a +3.00 D add. Eighty-five percent of patients experienced significant improvement in diplopia symptoms after monovision correction, and none of the 20 cases withdrew from the study. Patients with small-angle diplopia are not good candidates for surgery due to the risk of overcorrection. Traditional noninvasive management with prisms should remain the first option due to the achievement of binocularity, but it does not work for all patients. Monovision correction with glasses, contact lenses, and IOLs are all potential modalities for diplopia management. For more discussion, see the section "Monovision to Correct Diplopia" in Chapter 5.

3.4 Laser Vision Correction Monovision

The customary goal of corneal laser vision correction is often stated as to reduce or eliminate the need for glasses and contact lenses. The two most common surgeries for laser vision correction for patients age 40 and above are to correct both eyes for distance or for monovision. A nomogram for near addition, with the degree of anisometropia increasing from approximately -1.25 D for a 40-year-old patient up to -2.50 D for a 65-year-old patient, has been used for laser vision correction monovision.[16,17]

Success rates for monovision laser correction range from 72 to 97.6%.[8,9] A comprehensive MEDLINE review[18] of 31 qualified studies by Arba Mosquera and Alió found that laser correction for monovision provides excellent distance and near uncorrected acuities, with a 17% retreatment and a 5% reversal rate.

In the study by Braun et al,[8] they found that LASIK monovision correction represents a viable and increasingly popular method of correcting presbyopic and prepresbyopic patients. Crossed monovision, correcting the dominant eye for near, could be applied successfully to appropriately chosen patients. The distance vision eye in monovision patients had a lower tolerance for residual refractive error and required a higher rate of enhancements.

Reilly et al[19] reported a success rate of 97.6% (success was defined as not needing to reverse the monovision, distance vision 20/25 or better, and near vision J2 or better) in 82 patients with myopic LASIK. There were 6 enhancements in the near eyes (7%) and 17 enhancements in the distance vision eyes (21%). This difference was statistically significant ($p = 0.007$). Thirty patients underwent a contact lens trial of monovision before LASIK, and none of those patients elected monovision reversal. There were 52 patients who did not undergo a contact lens monovision trial before LASIK monovision, and 2 of those patients underwent monovision reversal.

Creation of a possible multifocal corneal contour with LASIK may also contribute to the higher success rate. Good distance correction of the dominant eye, good blur suppression without strong sighting preference, reasonable postoperative anisometropia, lack of significant phoria, and relatively preserved stereovision are the main factors to achieve success, but it is not without compromises. A study by Alarcón et al[20] enrolled 25 patients (50 eyes) with a mean age of 49.3 ± 4.5 (SD) years. Postoperatively, more than 90% of patients had a binocular uncorrected distance and near visual acuity of 0.0 LogMAR or better, although the contrast sensitivity function diminished, especially in the nondominant eye. Stereoacuity was significantly worse in all patients ($p < 0.001$). In all eyes, the mean objective light scatter index value increased postoperatively, but not significantly ($p > 0.05$).

3.5 Conductive Keratoplasty

Conductive keratoplasty (CK) is an in-office procedure for the correction of hyperopia, hyperopic astigmatism, and presbyopia. The procedure uses controlled release of high-frequency, low-energy electric current to generate thermal energy in the cornea and cause corneal steepening by stromal collagen shrinkage. One of the most common approaches using CK was to make the nondominant eye myopic for near vision and reading. The term "blended vision" was introduced by Refractec, a company founded in 1993 to develop and market the CK system, and to distinguish the CK system from traditional monovision; but at the insistence of the U.S. Food and Drug Administration (FDA), Refractec dropped "blended vision" from its labeling.[21] Instead, Refractec used the term NearVision CK. It serves as an alternative to laser-based refractive surgery with essentially no intraoperative or postoperative complications. The U.S. FDA approved CK in 2002.[21] Mendez and colleagues were likely the first to use the procedure in 1993.[22]

At the 6-month follow-up of a 1-year FDA study in 2004, McDonald et al found that the procedure appeared to be very safe and effective in producing functional visual acuity and patient satisfaction was similar to that of monovision LASIK.[23] The main downside of this procedure is its durability. A few years after the procedure, the steepening of the cornea shows some regression of effect.

A study by Stahl[24] supported the long-term safety, efficacy, and stability of CK in the unilateral treatment of presbyopia performed in the nondominant eye of 10 near-plano presbyopic patients to improve their near vision. The preoperative mean near vision without correction was J10, but 3 years after CK, the mean near uncorrected visual acuity (UCVA) was J3. The mean manifest refraction spherical equivalent (MRSE) at 3 years was -1.06 ± 0.81 D, which represented a 0.25 D loss of effect from that at 1 year. They also reported a +0.25 D change in MRSE in the dominant untreated eyes during a period of 3 years. This change is not statistically different from the CK-treated eyes during the 3-year postoperative period. Seventy-eight percent of eyes reported binocular distance UCVA 20/20 or better and near UCVA J3 or better. In their cohort, no eye lost best spectacle-corrected visual acuity (BSCVA) or had induced cylinder greater than or equal to 0.75 D. They also reported stable keratometry with 45.09 D compared to 45.08 D reported at 3 and 1 year postoperatively.

A study done by Ayoubi et al compared the visual outcomes, complications, and patient satisfaction after femtosecond LASIK and CK in a retrospective consecutive single-surgeon comparative study in private laser clinics in the United Kingdom and found that there were 3% and 50% retreatment rates after femtosecond LASIK and CK ($p < 0.0001$), respectively.[25] The satisfaction rate in a 12-month follow-up survey noted 62.5% in the femtosecond LASIK group, and 34.4% in the CK group reported being satisfied ($p = 0.02$). The study concluded that femtosecond LASIK monovision provided stable correction with less induced astigmatism and higher-order aberrations. Eyes with CK monovision had regression and induced astigmatism.

CK was also used in pseudophakic patients to create monovision.[26] Ye et al evaluated the visual outcomes of CK for relief of symptomatic presbyopia of pseudophakia with monofocal intraocular lens implantation in 27 eyes of 27 patients. Twelve months after CK, the binocular UNVA was significantly improved from LogMAR 0.88 ± 0.16 preoperatively to LogMAR 0.30 ± 0.13 ($p < 0.05$); the binocular UDVA and best spectacle corrected visual acuity remained unchanged; manifest refractive spherical equivalent was significantly reduced from preoperative 0.01 ± 0.68 D to postoperative -1.68 ± 0.39 D ($p < 0.05$).

References

[1] Weakley DR. The association between anisometropia, amblyopia, and binocularity in the absence of strabismus. Trans Am Ophthalmol Soc. 1999; 97:987–1021

[2] Parks MM. The 1999 Gunter K. von Noorden visiting professorship lecture. Monovsion: the case for two binocular vision systems. Binocul Vis Strabismus Q. 2000; 15(1):13–16

[3] Evans BJ. Monovision: a review. Ophthalmic Physiol Opt. 2007; 27(5):417–439

[4] Westsmith RA. Uses of a monocular contact lens. Am J Ophthalmol. 1958; 46(1, Pt 1):78–81

[5] Fonda G. Presbyopia corrected with single vision spectacles or corneal lenses in preference to bifocal corneal lenses. Trans Ophthalmol Soc Aust. 1966; 25:78–80

[6] Harris MG, Sheedy JE, Gan CM. Vision and task performance with monovision and diffractive bifocal contact lenses. Optom Vis Sci. 1992; 69(8):609–614

[7] Back AP, Holden BA, Hine NA. Correction of presbyopia with contact lenses: comparative success rates with three systems. Optom Vis Sci. 1989; 66(8):518–525

[8] Braun EH, Lee J, Steinert RF. Monovision in LASIK. Ophthalmology. 2008; 115(7):1196–1202

[9] Jain S, Ou R, Azar DT. Monovision outcomes in presbyopic individuals after refractive surgery. Ophthalmology. 2001; 108(8):1430–1433

[10] Jain S, Arora I, Azar DT. Success of monovision in presbyopes: review of the literature and potential applications to refractive surgery. Surv Ophthalmol. 1996; 40(6):491–499

[11] Bujak MC, Leung AK, Kisilevsky M, Margolin E. Monovision correction for small-angle diplopia. Am J Ophthalmol. 2012; 154(3):586–592.e2

[12] London R. Monovision correction for diplopia. J Am Optom Assoc. 1987; 58(7):568–570

[13] Migneco MK. Alleviating vertical diplopia through contact lenses without the use of prism. Eye Contact Lens. 2008; 34(5):297–298

[14] Lubkin V, Stollerman H, Linksz A. Stereopsis in monocular aphakia with spectacle correction. Am J Ophthalmol. 1966; 61(2):273–276

[15] Greenbaum S. Monovision pseudophakia. J Cataract Refract Surg. 2002; 28(8):1439–1443

[16] Goldberg DB. Laser in situ keratomileusis monovision. J Cataract Refract Surg. 2001; 27(9):1449–1455

[17] Goldberg DB. Comparison of myopes and hyperopes after laser in situ keratomileusis monovision. J Cataract Refract Surg. 2003; 29(9):1695–1701

[18] Arba Mosquera S, Alió JL. Presbyopic correction on the cornea. Eye Vis (Lond). 2014; 1:5

[19] Reilly CD, Lee WB, Alvarenga L, Caspar J, Garcia-Ferrer F, Mannis MJ. Surgical monovision and monovision reversal in LASIK. Cornea. 2006; 25(2):136–138

[20] Alarcón A, Anera RG, Villa C, Jiménez del Barco L, Gutierrez R. Visual quality after monovision correction by laser in situ keratomileusis in presbyopic patients. J Cataract Refract Surg. 2011; 37(9):1629–1635

[21] Azar DT, Gatinel D, Hoang-Xuan T. Refractive Surgery. 2nd ed. Philadelphia, PA: Mosby; 2006

[22] Du TT, Fan VC, Asbell PA. Conductive keratoplasty. Curr Opin Ophthalmol. 2007; 18(4):334–337

[23] McDonald MB, Durrie D, Asbell P, Maloney R, Nichamin L. Treatment of presbyopia with conductive keratoplasty: six-month results of the 1-year United States FDA clinical trial. Cornea. 2004; 23(7):661–668

[24] Stahl JE. Conductive keratoplasty for presbyopia: 3-year results. J Refract Surg. 2007; 23(9):905–910

[25] Ayoubi MG, Leccisotti A, Goodall EA, McGilligan VE, Moore TC. Femtosecond laser in situ keratomileusis versus conductive keratoplasty to obtain monovision in patients with emmetropic presbyopia. J Cataract Refract Surg. 2010; 36(6):997–1002

[26] Ye P, Xu W, Tang X, et al. Conductive keratoplasty for symptomatic presbyopia following monofocal intraocular lens implantation. Clin Experiment Ophthalmol. 2011; 39(5):404–411

4 Pseudophakic Monovision

Abstract

The hole-in-card dominance test, the plus lens mimic test, and the cover/uncover test are essential tests to have high success in pseudophakic monovision. Contact lens trial is not necessary for most routine cases. Compromised fine stereopsis, decreased uncorrected distance vision of the near eye, and lack of guaranteed 100% glasses independence are three key topics for consultation with prospective IOL monovision patients. Anisometropia of 1.00 to 1.50 D works well for the majority of patients with good binocular stereopsis and contrast, although they may have more chance of needing backup readers than full monovision at the 1.75 D or more level. Conventional IOL monovision is still preferred, although crossed IOL monovision also works well as long as the anisometropia level is mild to modest and contraindications are avoided. Crossed IOL monovision is commonly applied in many situations, such as when the first eye refractive target is missed.

If a patient has a history of monovision and is doing well without problems, keep the same pattern regardless of the dominant eye test. Operating on the priority goal eye first will give the surgeon two chances to reach the priority refractive target in case the first operated eye refraction target is missed. Ocular contraindications of IOL monovision are mainly EOM related. IOL monovision does not work well if a patient has systemic contraindications. Avoiding contraindications is one of the three keys to IOL monovision success. Monovision knowledge and skills are helpful and sometimes essential for the success of premium IOL refractive cataract surgery.

Keywords: preoperative tests for pseudophakic monovision, preoperative consultation for IOL monovision, astigmatism and monovision, anisometropia level and monovision, crossed monovision, monovision contraindications, multifocal IOL and monovision, Symfony IOL and monovision, accommodating IOL and monovision

4.1 Introduction

The concept of one stone to kill two birds is at the core of using intraocular lens (IOL) monovision for the management of presbyopia in cataract patients. The fundamental component of monovision is increasing the depth of focus while maintaining acceptable stereovision. Binocular depth of focus is associated with the sum of two monocular ranges of clear vision, spanning from the near focal point to the far focal point. It is quite reasonable to consider a certain amount of power difference between the two eyes in terms of the postoperative refractive target when the surgeon chooses an IOL implant. This is done with the hope that postoperatively the patient will not need spectacles for daily activities or will decrease any dependence on spectacles. In conventional monovision, typically, the dominant eye is chosen for distance vision and the nondominant eye for near. The reverse pattern, dominant eye for near and nondominant eye for far, is called crossed monovision.

Boerner and Thrasher[1] were the first authors to describe a pseudophakic monovision study in the literature. They retrospectively analyzed the postoperative rate of glasses use in 100 patients with bilateral posterior chamber IOL (PCIOL) monovision. The number of patients needing to wear bifocals postoperatively declined by half with this technique.

There are numerous studies in the literature that demonstrate the impressive success of pseudophakic monovision. Patient satisfaction/spectacle freedom has been approximately 80% or more,[2,3,4,5,6,7] while overwhelmingly most postoperative cataract patients will need to wear reading glasses (160 out of 169 patients) if both eyes were targeted at plano to –0.50 D spherical equivalent.[8]

For the sake of discussion without confusion, we would recommend the following classification for pseudophakic monovision in terms of focal length separation between the two eyes:

- Mini (sometimes referred to as micro or nano), –0.50 to –0.75 D.
- Modest (sometimes referred to as medium), –1.00 to –1.5 D.
- Full (sometimes referred to as traditional or classical), –1.75 to –2.5 D.

4.2 Preoperative Tests for Pseudophakic Monovision

The first eye dominance test recorded was probably by Porta in the sixteenth century, but it did not seem to get much attention until the 1920s.[9,10,11] In the mid-1920s, Sheard[10,11] proposed not to weaken the dominant sighting eye in order to maintain balance. He believed that the object looked at is sighted by the dominant eye in its own line of vision, while the nondominant eye then has to converge until binocular single vision occurs. Thus, there is dominance of one member in each pair, whether we refer to the hands, the feet, or the eyes. He proposed that if the patient has a strongly dominant eye, the clinician should leave the acuity slightly better in this eye than in the fellow eye. Otherwise, the patient may experience some discomfort. If there is no significant eye dominance, then we should try to achieve equal function in both eyes. If prism is needed, it should mostly be placed in front of the weaker eye. These refraction rules proposed by early clinicians such as Sheard were designed to enhance binocular function and lessen asthenopia. They laid out the importance of the role of dominance in monovision. Despite these rules, crossed IOL monovision can still work well within a certain range.[4,12]

Preoperative dominant eye tests for monovision can be divided basically into two groups. One is a motor sighting dominance test and one is a sensory dominance test. The patient is forced to choose one eye over the other in the motor sighting dominance test, while the patient is asked about balance and perceptual preference in the sensory ocular dominance test. The motor sighting dominance test contains stereo-objects with a disparity beyond Panum's area, while sensory ocular dominance, also referred to as ocular prevalence, is determined using stereo-targets imaged within Panum's area.[13]

4.2.1 Commonly Used Sighting Dominance Tests

Hole-in-Card (5 × 9 Inch Card with a Central 1.25-Inch Hole, NearVision CK)

- Done with distance glasses or without glasses, whichever provides better distance vision for the patient.
- Choose a small target at the end of the room, about 10 to 20 feet away.
- The patient extends both arms and holds the card with the thumb and the index finger in *both* hands.
- The patient is asked to keep both eyes open and to align the hole to the target.
- The examiner covers each eye in turn. The eye aligned with the hole and the target is the sighting dominant eye.

Finger Pointing

- Done with distance glasses or without glasses, whichever provides better distance vision for the patient.
- The patient extends the dominant arm.
- Ask the patient to choose a small target at the end of the room, about 10 to 20 feet away. With both eyes open, have the index finger point at the target.
- Close one eye and then the other. The eye that aligns the index finger and the target is the dominant eye.
- Given the fact that only one arm is used to point at the target, the concern for this test is the potential influence of the hand sidedness. A better way[14] might be to use both extended arms holding a pencil. The patient is asked to align the tip of the pencil with the distance target and the observer occludes each eye alternatively to find out which eye is aligned with the target. The eye that remains in line with the target is the sighting dominant eye.

Finger Hole

- Done with distance glasses or without glasses, whichever provides better distance vision.
- The patient extends both arms and brings both hands together, forming a small hole by crossing the thumbs and index fingers.
- Choose a small target at the end of the room, about 10 to 20 feet away. With both eyes open, view the target through the small hole.
- The examiner covers each eye in turn. The eye aligned with the hole and the target is the sighting dominant eye.

Camera or Kaleidoscope

- Most people automatically use their dominant eye when looking through a camera or a kaleidoscope eyepiece.
- The patient is asked to hold the camera with *both* hands and bring the camera to the face.
- The eye using the camera is the dominant eye.

Mirror Test

- The patient looks into a small mirror, held at 20 cm, containing a 1-inch diameter circle.
- This results in an optical target distance of 40 cm. The patient sights his or her nose within the mirror.
- Ocular dominance is determined by identifying the sighting eye by alternating eye closure.

4.2.2 Commonly Used Sensory Dominance Tests

Compared to the motor sighting dominant eye test, sensory rivalry is not primarily viewed as a tool for measuring ocular dominance, but rather for studying the neural correlation of visual perception. Sensory dominance may occur when there is a difference in the two retinal images that could lead to rivalry or some binocular interaction. For example, there may be differences in image clarity, brightness, or color. Based on these differences, the visual system might find it easier to suppress one eye than the other, or to favor one eye over the other. Some other sensory-based tests use a binocular rivalry target or stereodisparate objects to evaluate the magnitude of sensory dominance quantitatively. This potentially will be the future direction of preoperative monovision tests because it can be measured quantitatively.

Distance Sensory Dominance with a Plus Lens

Consider a person who requires a + 1.50 D add. Let the person, with distance glasses or no glasses, whichever gives better distance vision, fixate on the far visual acuity chart binocularly and introduce a + 1.50 D lens over the right and then left eye. See if the patient notices any difference in the clarity of the letters binocularly when either the right or the left eye is blurred. If, for example, the binocular visual acuity is better and also the patient feels more comfortable and natural when the left eye is blurred, it is the nondominant eye. Blurring the dominant eye (in this case, the right) is more disagreeable. That is, the patient prefers to have the right eye unblurred at far.

Near Sensory Dominance with Plus Lens

With the patient's current distance glasses, or most recent manifest refraction in a trial frame, a clip-on + 1.50 D lens or a single + 1.50 D free lens is placed in front of one eye and then the other eye. The patient is asked to read for a few minutes and then asked to tell the observer if he/she feels better balanced and more natural if the plus lens is over the right eye or the left eye. If the patient feels more comfortable when the plus lens is over the right eye, the right eye is dominant for near and the left eye is nondominant for near. Near sensory dominance with a plus lens is not commonly used in clinic practice session.

Worth Four Dot Test at Near and Far

The Worth Four Dot (W4D) test can be used to evaluate fusion function as well as sensory dominance status. For the sensory function evaluation, the patient views the target wearing red-green glasses. The patient is asked to tell what color appears for the white dot. If the white appears to be reddish, then the eye behind the red filter is the sensory dominant eye, and if the white dot appears to be greenish, then the eye behind the green filter is the sensory dominant eye. It is not always that straightforward, since sometimes the patient will tell you the color is "orange" or they are "unable to tell." Of note, during the distance test, the patient should wear his or her regular distance glasses if the patient needs distance glasses for driving or watching TV; otherwise, the number and color of the target dots can be hard to distinguish for those who need a significant refractive correction. Visual acuity and cataract density can influence this test. The cloudy lens can have a similar impact as adding a neutral density filter. Some projection distance W4D tests can be too small for cataract patients. That means the visual angle of the target dots require 20/20 or 20/25 vision; if acuity is less, this may result in a false-negative evaluation. Clinically, this test is mainly used for fusion function rather than for a dominance test. For example, when the clinician is evaluating a monovision candidate suspected of having amblyopia or monofixation syndrome, and if the patient is able to see all four dots at distance, this tells the clinician that the patient is more likely a good candidate for IOL monovision. However, if the patient can see only three dots or fewer at distance, that can be either due to a fusion issue, as in amblyopia and monofixation, or due to poor vision from dense cataract or other ocular pathology.

4.2.3 Monovision Plus Lens Mimic Test

The plus lens test has dual functions in monovision evaluation, one being what we discussed earlier—distance sensory dominance with a plus lens—and the other being the monovision mimic test.

The monovision plus lens mimic test has been called many different names: the tolerance test, interocular defocus threshold test, myopic defocus threshold test, or blur tolerance test.

There are several ways to do this simulating preoperative monovision mimic test. It gives the patient a chance to experience the mimicked monovision status.

4.2.4 Tolerance Test[15] of William Maloney

This is a very meticulous step-by-step test and can yield very detailed information. It works very well but it takes much more time than other tests for the same purpose.

4.2.5 Drs. Finkelman and Barrett Use a More Straightforward Test[6]

Place the distance correction in a trial frame. A + 1.00 D lens is used to demonstrate the predicted outcome of monovision. In their study, the first eye was already operated on with good distance vision and the second eye waiting to have surgery was to be the near eye.

4.2.6 Siepser Blur Tolerance Test

A beautiful demonstration can be found on YouTube by searching "Siepser Blur Tolerance Test." The value of this test is that it enables a dynamic but still easy-to-perform test for both the patient and the examiner.

4.2.7 The Following Is What We Have Been Using for the Past Few Years at F. Z.'s Office

Each patient receives a plus lens test, which has two different meanings: the first is the mimic test where the plus lens with a magnetic clip (▶ Fig. 4.1, ▶ Fig. 4.2, ▶ Fig. 4.3, ▶ Fig. 4.4) is placed in front of the nondominant eye (decided by hole-in-card). By doing this, the patient will have a chance to understand that the distance vision of the near eye is not very clear although the reading vision is better. The patient will need to tell the examiner if he or she finds this condition acceptable.

The second part of the plus lens test is the sensory dominance test with a magnetic clip-on plus lens (▶ Fig. 4.1, ▶ Fig. 4.2, ▶ Fig. 4.3, ▶ Fig. 4.4) placed in front of each eye monocularly when the patient wears their regular distance glasses, if there was no significantly improved vision with a new manifest refraction (▶ Fig. 4.3), or in front of the new manifest lenses placed in a trial frame for distance if there was improvement with the new manifest (▶ Fig. 4.4).

The sensory dominance test with the plus lens is tested for distance where the patient is asked to

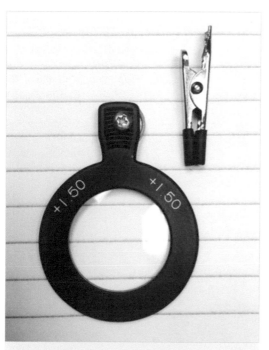

Fig. 4.1 Plus lens 1.50 D with a magnetic clip.

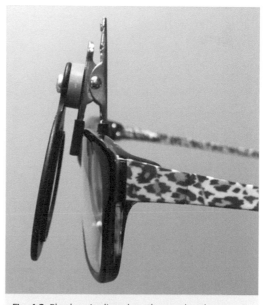

Fig. 4.2 Plus lens is clipped on the regular glasses.

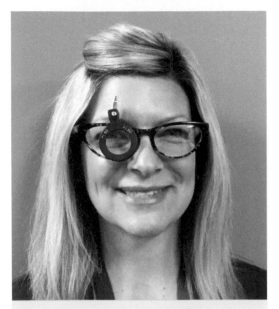

Fig. 4.3 Plus lens tested with her regular glasses.

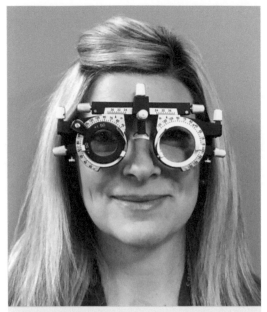

Fig. 4.4 Plus lens tested with trial frame when the new refraction offers better vision.

binocularly look at the distance visual acuity chart at 20 feet while the plus lens is placed in front of each eye monocularly. The patient is asked to report in front of which eye the plus lens is placed when he or she has overall better binocular vision and feels more natural and comfortable. If the patient feels better when the plus lens is in front of the right eye, then the *left* eye is the sensory dominant eye since the patient feels more uncomfortable when the dominant left eye is blurred due to the extra plus lens.

Each patient should also be allowed a few minutes of walking in the hallway while wearing the plus lens to test comfort and feeling of balance. If the patient does not like mimicked monovision and/or balance sensation, no monovision will be offered.

4.2.8 Dominance Test Interpretations and Variations

The results from different sighting dominance tests for the same person can vary. For example, the hole-in-card shows OD as dominant, but the camera shows OS. It would be interesting to find out if these patients have relatively weak dominance or no clear preference for either the right or left eye. It is possible that these patients have a better prognosis for success with IOL monovision,

regardless of whether it is conventional or crossed monovision, than those patients with strong dominance for one eye. Patients with alternating dominance (no sighting preference) have better interocular blur suppression, which is another predictive factor for monovision success, while those with a strong sighting preference have reduced blur suppression, decreased binocular depth of focus, and higher monovision failure rates.[16,17,18,19,20,21,22,23] For alternating sighting dominance patients, the binocular depth of focus is almost equal to the sum of monocular depths of focus, but in those with strong sighting dominance, the binocular image becomes blurred as the object moves from the dominant eye's clear range to the nondominant eye's clear range, and thus the binocular depth of focus in those patients is much less than the sum of the monocular depths of focus.[21] Extremely strong dominance examples can be seen in amblyopia and monofixation syndromes, where the suppression for the stronger eye is very difficult, and that is the reason why those patients do not do well with monovision.

Sighting dominance is not fixed, but rather plastic and fluid, even with the same testing method. More than half a century ago, Charnwood[24] had already noted that sighting dominance changes when the refractive correction changes. That is probably the reason why, in most situations, crossed monovision works as well as conventional monovision. Based on 10 ocularly healthy young patients, Khan and Crawford[25] were able to demonstrate that in a reach-grasp task for targets within the binocular visual field, patients switched between left and right eye dominance depending on horizontal gaze angle. The sighting dominance can even change as the person looks at different places in the visual field and even at different times.[16]

In the aging population, the vision and the refractive status can change significantly as a consequence of cataract formation and refractive index change. It is not rare to notice that sighting dominance changes due to cataract density change and due to refractive status change or vision change. A recent study by Schwartz and Yatziv[26] noted eye dominance changed after cataract surgery due to improved vision: of the 33 patients included, 7 patients (21.2%) had a change in ocular dominance from nondominance to dominance due to improved vision.

The hole-in-card test is the most popular motor sighting dominance test, while the plus lens is the most popular sensory dominance test in cataract surgery IOL monovision clinical settings. Between the two types of tests, there is no simple conclusion in terms of correlation. That means the motor sighting dominant eye is not always the sensory dominant eye and is not always the better vision eye.[13,14,16,27,28,29,30,31,32]

A prospective study with 51 emmetropic patients, aged 18 to 60 years, done by Seijas et al[14] compared multiple tests of motor sighting dominance and sensory ocular dominance. Patients were divided into two groups: 18 to 35 years old (26 patients) and 35 to 60 years old (25 patients). In the motor sighting test group, hole-in-card, kaleidoscope, point-a-finger, and convergence near point tests were evaluated. Hole-in-card and kaleidoscope tests had the most certain results, while the rest had more variation. There was no good agreement among these tests either. In the sensory test group, + 1.00 D lens, W4D test, polarized test, Haidinger's test, and distance stereo test were evaluated. Plus 1.00 D lens was found to have the most certain results, while the rest had more variation. Similar to the motor sighting tests, very poor correlation existed among the different tests in the sensory group. The agreement of motor sighting dominant eye with hole-in-card with + 1.00 D lens sensory ocular dominance tests was only 58% in young patients (15 of 26) and 40% (10 of 25) in older patients. The agreement among other motor and sensory tests was much lower. It

was apparent that most of the studied patients did not show clear ocular dominance, because the results were quite variable and little correlation was found among the tests. Most people have a constantly alternating balance between both eyes. This study result suggests that most patients may do well with IOL monovision. Those who do not tolerate monovision might be those who have strong and clear ocular dominance or those with contraindications for monovision. It is true that the main emphasis of preoperative monovision tests is not to find out which eye is dominant, right versus left, but it is to find out who might not be able to tolerate surgically created monovision. For example, those who have the same eye dominant for both distance and near may have clear and strong ocular dominance and therefore may have a high chance of failure, because monovision forces them to change the viewing distance.

A study[31] by Suttle et al was in agreement with the study by Seijas et al.[14] Generally speaking, ocular dominance shows poor agreement between methods within individuals. Those experimental studies correlate well with our clinical practice. They appear to explain why overwhelmingly most crossed IOL monovision patients do as well as conventional IOL monovision patients, as long as contraindications are avoided and the anisometropia level is kept at a mini or modest level.

An experimental study using a stereoscope in 60 new contact lens–wearing monovision patients by Collins and Goode[22] demonstrated that when the sensory rivalry dominant eye matched the sighting dominant eye, blur suppression and monovision were better. Our own study of 10-year follow-up IOL monovision patients supports that phenomenon: among 45 IOL monovision patients who had both tests, 24 out of 45 were matched between hole-in-card and plus lens test at distance; 18 out of 45 were unmatched and 3 out of 45 were uncertain. The matched group had better results, especially in satisfaction and nighttime driving evaluation with statistically significant p-values.

We do not have an easy way to quantitatively measure rivalry sensory dominance in our busy clinic. The most commonly used test seems to be the plus lens. If the same eye is dominant in the rivalry sensory test for both far and near, that patient probably has a strong rivalry sensory dominance and is likely to have more difficulty in blur suppression and may have a high chance of monovision failure. Full monovision should be avoided in those patients. It would be valuable to have rivalry sensory tests for all prospective IOL monovision patients, to objectively and quantitatively measure the strength of rivalry dominance, although we still do not know how much impact dense cataracts have in terms of reliability and accuracy.

Handa et al[18] studied 20 IOL monovision patients; 16 of them were successful and 4 of them were unsuccessful with a follow-up of more than 6 months after cataract surgery. The study was able to quantitatively measure sensory dominance and suggested that strong sensory ocular dominance has a direct negative impact on the success of IOL monovision. The study was done when the patients already had IOLs in their eyes, so it would likely be quite different if measured preoperatively with the cloudy cataract. Strong ocular dominance may have a high chance of monovision failure since it is harder for those patients to have blur suppression. When the nondominant eye is fixing, the dominant eye will not easily suppress the blur, which will produce visual stress on binocular balance.

Ooi and He did a well-designed experiment with 32 patients who had equal vision of at least 20/20 in each eye, good stereoacuity of at least 40 seconds of arc, and normal color vision with no previous history of ocular disease or surgery.[30] The hypothesis was if the inferiority of the nondominant eye is solely due to a weakness in its monocular channel before the convergence of binocular information, its other visual functions, such as contrast sensitivity and suprathreshold brightness judgment, when measured monocularly, should also be inferior relative to those functions in the dominant eye. However, if interocular imbalance caused by sensory eye dominance is largely attributable to processes at the binocular visual stage, at which the information from the two eyes has combined, the monocular information retained in the monocular channels should be equally preserved. Hence, the contrast sensitivity and suprathreshold brightness judgment functions measured in each eye should be the same. By adjusting the strength of the stimulus to find the neutral point between the two eyes, rather than adding neutral density filters, the study was able to quantitatively measure sensory dominance of each eye. That study had quite a few interesting findings:

1. There was no correlation between the sighting dominant eye and sensory dominant eye.
2. The monocular contrast sensitivity test did not directly correlate with the motor sighting dominant eye test result or sensory dominance test.
3. Monocular brightness perception did have a nearly significant relation with the sensory

dominance test ($p = 0.0512$), suggesting that there was a statistically meaningful relationship between interocular imbalance (sensory dominance) and monocular brightness perception.
4. Monocular brightness perception did not have direct correlation with the sighting dominance test.
5. Sensory dominance could not be predicted from refractive status.
6. Based on the above findings, their main conclusion was that the sensory dominance is largely attributable to processes in binocular, not monocular channels, since monocular input of either contrast or brightness did not correlate with sensory dominance.

4.2.9 Is a Preoperative Monovision Mimic Test Necessary?

Our own study reviewed all cataract surgery charts from January 2005 to December 2014 at F. Z.'s office. Based on preoperative plus lens tests, patients were divided into tested and untested. Parameters at their last office visit were analyzed including visual acuity, satisfaction, spectacle independence, real-life gross depth perception issues, and nighttime driving difficulties when they did not wear glasses. In total, 359 cases were qualified (30 passed away, 87 lost contact during 10 years) and 194 patients were enrolled with de-identified surveys, 100 with the plus lens test, and 94 without the test. Average postoperative follow-up was 34 months in the tested group and 36 months in the untested group. Mean anisometropia was 1.38 D in the tested group and 1.21 D in the untested group ($p = 0.006$). Both groups had very high satisfaction of 95% or above. That study suggested that a preoperative mimic test may not be necessary to achieve high patient satisfaction in IOL monovision as long as a good preoperative monovision consultation was provided.

The preoperative monovision mimic test has two meanings: one being a sensory dominance test for the clinician, and one being a mimic test for the patient. First, we know sighting and sensory dominance do not always match. Second, we usually choose the sighting dominant eye for the distance eye and the nondominant eye for near, and this has been the convention. The test has unique merit in giving the patient a mimicked experience of one eye for far and one eye for near; plus, the test is brief and can be done by a technician. This test indirectly tells each prospective monovision patient the fact that monovision is not perfect, but it is a compromise. Therefore, our recommendation is to do this test for every prospective IOL monovision patient. If the patient does not like the sensation when sitting or walking with the presence of a plus lens, then it is not a good idea to offer IOL monovision to this patient, even if there are no other contraindications. The plus lens test may not be absolutely necessary and critical,[5,33] but it is advisable as part of the preoperative consultation.

4.2.10 Is a Contact Lens Trial Test Necessary for IOL Monovision?

Many surgeons do a contact lens trial, mainly in patients being evaluated for monovision laser refractive surgery,[34,35,36,37,38] with a very understandable rationale: to be cautious since surgically induced monovision is hard to reverse if a patient is not a good candidate.

Reilly and colleagues[37] reviewed 82 patients who elected to undergo surgical monovision with LASIK between 2000 and 2003. Thirty of the 82 underwent a contact lens trial of monovision before the surgery and none of them elected monovision reversal. There were 52 patients who did not undergo a contact lens trial prior to the surgery; 2 of them underwent monovision reversal. These findings were similar to a study done by Goldberg,[36] who found that 5 of 114 monovision patients who elected to have their monovision reversed had not had a trial of contact lens monovision or a history of contact lens monovision correction. Although it may seem intuitive to offer patients contemplating monovision a trial of contact lens monovision correction, some might argue that the reversal rate is so low that a trial is not warranted.

IOL monovision is different from laser vision–induced monovision. Without a contact lens trial, the IOL success rate can still be very high. A study by Greenbaum[5] with 140 IOL monovision patients demonstrated a 92% (129 patients) success rate. There was no contact lens trial performed prior to the decision for monovision. Of note, for the patients in that study, the near vision eye was aimed at −2.75 D and the distance vision eye was aimed at emmetropia, although there was no average anisometropic level between the two eyes listed in the paper. Many other pseudophakic monovision studies, also with high patient satisfaction and spectacle independence rates, but lower levels of anisometropic level than 2.75 D, did not have contact lens trials prior to cataract surgery.[2,3,4,6,7,33,39,40]

In individuals with myopia or hyperopia without significant astigmatism, a contact lens trial should be relatively easy. However, contact lens trials can be difficult or not realistic if there is severe astigmatism, or if the patient is unable to use a lens due to a systemic or ocular condition or advanced age, if the patient does not want to go through the process, or if the cataract is dense with very poor vision. The process of a contact lens trial itself can be difficult and it can be discouraging for most elderly patients if they never used contact lenses before.

For many years, when I (F. Z.) received questions from surgeons who had just started to do pseudophakic monovision, a frequent question was "is it necessary to have a contact lens trial prior to the surgery?" My answer was typically "It is reasonable, but not necessary." It is probably reasonable or even advisable to conduct a contact lens trial for those patients with demanding personalities, and those patients who are not willing to consider glasses after surgery if they are not able to tolerate postoperative IOL monovision. With dense cataracts and poor vision, the accuracy is questionable. The pseudophakic monovision patient population is clearly different from the laser vision correction monovision group. Among several thousand IOL monovision cases over two decades, I (F. Z.) have had only two patients who had a contact lens trial prior to decision-making. The first case was a psychiatrist who had a history of high myopia, retinal detachment, monofocal contact lens monovision 15 years earlier, and then multifocal contact lenses prior to cataract surgery. She was a candidate for either monofocal IOL monovision or multifocal IOLs since she had monofocal contact lens monovision and multifocal contact lenses before and was happy in both situations. My first choice was monofocal IOL monovision rather than multifocal IOLs due to her relatively young age, imperfect macula on optical coherence tomography (OCT), high level of corneal astigmatism (there was no combined multifocal IOL with toric IOL on the US market at that time), and her frequent need for nighttime driving. In order to make sure that IOL monovision would be her first option rather than a multifocal IOL, I had her go through a 2-week monofocal contact lens trial set by my optometrist colleague. She ended up as a happy IOL monovision patient. The second patient who had a contact lens trial already had a modest level of anisometropia IOL monovision, but she wanted to have full monovision with her near eye about −3.00 D to cover her reading. We typically discourage separating two eyes by more than 2.50 D, but that patient insisted on having 3.00 D anisometropia with a piggyback IOL, so a contact lens trial was ordered for her before the piggyback IOL decision. (See the case report "How Much Anisometropia Works Best?" later in this chapter.) Otherwise, without contact lens trials in two decades of practice, I only had to take two patients back to the operating room for a piggyback IOL, one to reverse monovision because I made a mistake in choosing the dominant eye for near (see the case report "Which Eye for Distance and Which Eye for Near?" later in this chapter) and one to enhance her from modest monovision to full monovision (see the case report "How Much Anisometropia Works Best?" later in this chapter). A contact lens trial for the first case would have been helpful to avoid the piggyback IOL, but not for the second case.

4.2.11 What Preoperative Tests Are Highly Recommended for Every IOL Monovision Patient?

There are many tests discussed in this section, and it can be difficult for a beginner to decide which ones are necessary.

Unintentional monovision happens when we miss refractive targets; but most such cases do not have any problem. Some clinicians routinely create monovision without any preoperative tests, but that approach can be risky and the success rate may not be as good as with testing and careful discussion. There is no clear-cut answer regarding which tests are necessary, but the following three tests are highly recommended, with good reason, for every prospective IOL monovision candidate.

Sighting Dominant Eye Tests

Most commonly used is the hole-in-card test.[14,31] One can also use a camera (a disposable camera costs only a few dollars and it is very handy to keep one in each room).

Without dominant eye tests and detailed past ocular history, monovision will have a higher rate of failure or, even worse, risk of postoperative deterioration of already compromised extraocular muscle (EOM) balance or even fixation switch diplopia (see details in the section "Fixation Switch Diplopia" later in the chapter).

Plus Lens Mimic Test

This test is also very simple and should be part of the preoperative consultation. A trained assistant can do this test well. As mentioned earlier, this test has two functions, one as a sensory dominance test for the clinician and one as a mimic tolerance test for the patient. With this mimic test, the patient will have an idea of what to expect as the postoperative status and it helps the patient to have realistic expectations. The patient will know that the uncorrected distance vision of the near eye will not be as good as the uncorrected distance vision of the distance eye. This test will also give you an idea if the patient has any issues in terms of anisometropic imbalance when sitting and walking.

Cover and Uncover Test

This test should not be missed. It tells you the basic EOM condition. It is also advisable to check all of the main gaze positions, including head tilt to right and left, since some congenital fourth nerve palsies can be asymptomatic. This assessment may be difficult or impossible if the cataract is very dense in one eye or both eyes. Sometimes, if the patient's vision is not good enough to allow fixation on the 20/400 chart, one can use a penlight as the target. Most IOL monovision candidates are able to perform this test. In those with very dense cataracts, either most do not have any desire to be spectacle independent (so no need to offer monovision) or they are not good candidates for IOL monovision, such as those with longstanding unilateral traumatic cataracts.

The above-mentioned three tests are highly recommended for every prospective IOL monovision candidate. Some tests are very helpful and become absolutely necessary in certain specific conditions. If you suspect a patient may have mild amblyopia or monofixation syndrome, or if cover and uncover testing reveals some phoria, then a stereo test, W4D test, and 4-diopter prism base-out test will be very helpful. (See further discussion in the sections "Potential Contraindications and Concerns for Pseudophakic Monovision" and "How to Detect Subtle Contraindications" later in the chapter.) If a patient with a history of successful multifocal contact lens use now wants to have IOL monovision, a monofocal contact lens trial is logical.

4.2.12 Summary of Preoperative Tests

The hole-in-card is the most commonly used sighting dominance test. The plus lens is the most commonly used sensory dominance and monovision mimic test for pseudophakic monovision. Sighting dominance test results are not fixed but can be plastic; they can change as vision or refractive status changes. A sighting dominance test prior to surgery is highly recommended since it can provide guidance in terms of conventional versus crossed IOL monovision. Plus lens sensory dominance and monovision mimic tests are valuable and advisable as part of preoperative consultation. The cover and uncover test should never be missed if it is possible to perform for IOL monovision candidates. It is reasonable to conduct a contact lens trial in specific cases, but it is not necessary for most routine cases.

4.3 What Are the Three Key Issues One Must Discuss with the Patient at the Preoperative Consultation?

Unintentional IOL monovision happens. Patients are typically happy with the unexpected result. Intentional IOL monovision is a premium refractive cataract surgery practice; to a certain degree, it is the same as use of a premium IOL. The patient has an expectation for quality vision as well as for spectacle independence. We cannot overestimate the importance of the preoperative consultation. The following three issues are highly recommended for full discussion, and accordingly, this discussion should be documented in the medical record.

4.3.1 There Will Be Decreased Fine Stereopsis

This is the main downside of monovision. We usually tell our patients: "You may need to wear readers when you try to thread a needle, but you should not expect issues with curbs, steps or stairs." Our 10-year review study demonstrated that only 0.5% of IOL monovision patients had to wear glasses all the time for depth perception, so the impact in real life is negligible.

4.3.2 The Distance Vision of the Near Eye Will Not Be As Sharp As the Distance Vision of the Far Eye

The is the main real-life compromise of monovision; while decreased stereovision is typically not noticeable, each patient needs to be informed

ahead of time. By far, this is the most common "negative" comment you will hear from your postoperative IOL monovision patients if you do not cover this in your preoperative consultation. Tell the patient that the near eye will still have good distance vision when it is needed, but may require a pair of backup glasses. Sometimes, the patient may forget what was discussed preoperatively; if so, just cover the near eye and ask the patient to read without glasses. This will make the patient appreciate the near eye function.

4.3.3 There Is No Guarantee of 100% Spectacle Freedom

Each candidate should understand that it is quite common to use backup glasses and occasionally some patients may need glasses all the time. It can vary as individual patient lifestyles and ocular conditions change in future years. Based on our own statistics, we now tell our patients: about 40% are completely glasses free, and 40% need some backup glasses only, such as for long duration reading of small print or nighttime driving. Around 15 to 20% need glasses for nighttime driving regardless of traffic or weather. These statistics are from our 10-year IOL monovision de-identified survey.

Besides the above three core concerns, the following list also needs the clinician's full attention. Without these, you are not providing a good consultation and the success rate and patient satisfaction can be compromised.

4.3.4 Expectation

Know what your patient wants before you consider your plan. A brief survey, either mailed to the patient's home before the office visit or completed by the patient/family in the office, will gather this information. The survey will tell you the patient's lifestyle, occupation, main hobbies, and desires. If a patient does not desire spectacle independence, there is no need to offer monovision or premium IOLs. Knowing this overall picture can efficiently direct your conversation during the busy office flow.

4.3.5 Personality and Priority

If a patient absolutely wants to be 100% glasses free and is not willing to consider backup glasses, then do not offer monovision or any premium IOL.

No one can offer a 100% guarantee. In my early career, I avoided offering IOL monovision to those marked as "perfectionist" on our survey sheet, but I have felt very comfortable for the last few years since I started using a "priority" strategy. (See details in the section "Which Eye to Operate upon First?" later in the chapter.) Basically, when this strategy is used, we have two chances to achieve the priority goal. By far, we do not need to change the preoperative plan if we have accurate biometry and deliver seamless surgery in the overwhelmingly majority of patients, but it is always a good idea to have a backup second chance. I do not recall any unhappy patient with a demanding personality since I have used this priority strategy for the last few years.

4.3.6 Main Hobbies

We ask our patients to list three main hobbies for which they wish to be glasses free. Based on this, we make our decision regarding what level of myopic defocus to choose for near. Of note, try to avoid using just the three main hobbies for decision-making. The case report in the section "How Much Anisometropia Works Best?" is a good example. That patient listed shopping, cooking, and biking, so modest IOL monovision was planned and delivered good vision, but the patient came back 2 years later wanting stronger reading power for her near eye, because I did not meet her "expectation" to be reading glasses free. I missed her occupation as a payroll worker and she did not like to wear glasses for her job (see details in the section "How Much Anisometropia Works Best?" later in the chapter).

4.3.7 Job or Previous Job

If a patient is a truck driver, you may wish to offer mini-monovision only. If a patient is a bookkeeper, the patient may want to have a priority for reading. We should avoid IOL monovision for a pilot.

4.3.8 Systemic Health Condition

Some systemic conditions are not ideal for IOL monovision, such as Parkinson's disease, myasthenia gravis, Graves' eye disease, and multiple sclerosis. All of these can potentially affect extraocular muscles and binocular function. We have them listed in our preoperative checklist to make sure we do not miss those contraindications.

4.3.9 Visual Confusion/Double Vision/Anxiety

Some patients may describe blurry or double images due to cataract or refractive changes as "double vision." A careful history and cover/uncover test should be able to detect the difference. Some patients are concerned whether they will have visual confusion when we set one eye for far and one eye for near. They should be reassured that they are much less likely to have those problems if we do a thorough preoperative screening. It is not rare for patients to have anxiety about monovision. These patients should be reassured. We should let them know that IOL monovision is reversible if the outcome is not desirable. The easiest correction is to wear glasses and very rarely do we need to use a piggyback IOL, IOL exchange, or laser vision correction. Patients with anxiety typically feel very relieved if we point out that contact lens monovision or laser vision monovision are the successful mainstay for precataract patients who do not like to use readers or bifocals.

4.3.10 Summary of Preoperative Consultation

Preoperative consultation is one of the three keys for IOL monovision success. Compromised fine stereopsis, decreased uncorrected distance vision of the near eye, and lack of a 100% glasses independence guarantee should be fully addressed for every IOL monovision candidate. Special attention should be paid to each patient's expectations, hobbies, job, and life style to customize for each individual's needs.

4.4 Astigmatism and IOL Monovision

Generally speaking, astigmatism has a negative impact on monovision performance and spectacle independence.[41,42,43] Astigmatism of 0.50 D or more in the dominant eye is less likely to yield very successful IOL monovision. The nondominant near vision eye, however, allows greater astigmatic tolerance. We have sometimes noted that patients still have good spectacle independence when the dominant eye has good distance vision and the nondominant near eye has residual astigmatism at the 1.00 to 1.50 D level. A study with added astigmatism in the spectacle plane in pseudophakic patients suggested that the allowable limit for astigmatism was in the range of 1.0 to 1.5 D for functional distance and near vision in both multi-focal and monofocal IOL patients.[44] Some studies suggested an acceptable amount of astigmatism of 1 D or less for IOL monovision.[2,3,33] A study by Greenbaum[5] reviewed 140 IOL monovision patients with a 92% (129 patients) success rate. Two diopters of preoperative astigmatism was listed as an exclusion criterion from enrollment for that study, although no postoperative residual astigmatism information was given in the paper.

A study documented the fact that distance acuity significantly deteriorated with uncorrected astigmatism, but near acuity improved with uncorrected myopic astigmatism and deteriorated with uncorrected hyperopic astigmatism.[45] How do we interpret this? Well, if you are presbyopic, put your correction for distance in a trial frame, and then test your reading. You will appreciate if you have an extra –1.00 D cylinder, but not + 1.00 D cylinder. The same study also suggested that together with the uncorrected myopic astigmatism, higher-order aberration improved near vision function in pseudophakic eyes.

If a patient wants to have IOL monovision but does not want to correct corneal astigmatism (for whatever reasons, usually due to the cost) and you find that the dominant eye has significant astigmatism which is not at or near your main incision location, you might better talk him or her out of monovision simply due to the potential effect of astigmatism on the final result. Although study[8] at Moorfields in 2009 suggested that the impact of astigmatism on reading-spectacle independence was smaller than the impact from hyperopia, meaning hyperopia causes more difficulty than astigmatism in terms of reading glasses, astigmatism is still a significant factor for glasses wear. As part of the Gutenberg Health study, a population-based cross-sectional study was conducted in the general population of Germany.[46] That study[46] had a total of 13,558 participants (49% female) with a mean age of 54.0 years (range, 35–74 years). The prevalence of refractive astigmatism (> 1.0 D) was 13.0% in right eyes and 12.0% in left eyes, and 85% of these participants wore distance spectacles.

Besides blurring the image, the effect induced by astigmatism may be due to meridional interocular suppression. This is more obvious for the dominant distance eye. The impact of astigmatism on the visual and optical system can also be associated with aniseikonia. Tolerance for aniseikonia varies from patient to patient. It is when the difference in image size or meridional distortions approaches the patient's tolerance that symptoms of aniseikonia become manifest and troublesome. Meridional distortions are more poorly tolerated, especially when they are oblique (not horizontal or vertical).[47]

Once surgery is done on both eyes, it is wise to observe the patient's function for a few months before considering surgical correction if there is significant residual astigmatism, especially if the residual astigmatism is in the near eye. (Typically, postoperative corneal topography is not billable, but we have found that it is important to do it on every patient who had a limbal relaxing incision [LRI] to find out the residual astigmatism, although we do not file a charge for it. It is also helpful in personalizing one's own LRI nomogram.) These patients often do well without further management while still maintaining reasonably good vision and satisfactory glasses independence. Simple LRI or laser vision correction can be used when the residual astigmatism needs correction. For toric implant patients, the intervention should be within the first few weeks to the first few months after the original surgery.

4.4.1 Summary of IOL Monovision and Astigmatism

Generally speaking, the less residual astigmatism the better, although it is quite reasonable to consider leaving a small amount with the rule cylinder due to aging change in postoperative years, especially in younger patients. Correction of astigmatism is critical for the dominant distance eye; residual astigmatism < 0.50 D seems to be essential to get good patient satisfaction and spectacle independence. The reading eye has greater astigmatism tolerance.

4.5 How Much Anisometropia Works Best?

We would recommend the following classification for Pseudophakic monovision in terms of focal length separation between the two eyes:
- Mini (sometimes referred to as micro or nano), –0.50 to –0.75 D.
- Modest (sometimes referred to as medium), –1.00 to –1.5 D.
- Full (sometimes referred to as traditional or classical), –1.75 to –2.5 D.

4.5.1 Mini and Modest Monovision Work Well for Most Patients

Spectacle independence after cataract surgery targeting bilateral emmetropia with monofocal IOLs is known to be low, in the range of 1 to 11%.[48] Another study noted that overwhelmingly most postoperative cataract patients needed to wear reading glasses (160 out of 169 patients) if both eyes were targeted for a plano to –0.50 D spherical equivalent.[8]

IOL monovision aims to create intentional anisometropia that increases depth of focus. How much focal length separation between the two eyes will be the best? There is no consensus regarding this concern. It varies depending on the clinician's experience and preferences as well as the patient's needs. Generally speaking, –1.25 to –1.50 D defocus is the preferred arrangement.[4,16,49,50,51,52,53,54] It is worth keeping in mind that pseudophakic accommodation can typically add 1 D to help near vision. More than 1.50 D can have a more noticeable impact on stereovision and contrast sensitivity.

The majority of mini-monovision patients (anisometropia less than 1.00 D) do well for far and intermediate focal distances, but usually need some help for reading, especially for prolonged periods. Labiris et al did a randomized study[39] with 38 mini-monovision patients and 37 multifocal IOL patients in 2014. For the monovision group, the dominant eye was aimed at –0.50 D and the nondominant eye was aimed at –1.25 D, with an average anisometropia level of 0.80 D. The spectacle-free rate for the monovision group was 31.4%. A study by Wilkins et al[33] found a 25.8% spectacle-free rate when the average power of the near eye was at –0.92 D.

High spectacle independence and patient satisfaction are achievable for most patients in both the conventional and crossed pseudophakic groups, which was demonstrated in a study by Zhang et al.[4] It is a common assumption that low anisometropia between the two eyes has a higher chance of needing glasses, but that study suggests that a modest anisometropia level (average about 1.15 D) can still achieve a high patient satisfaction rate (more than 95% were "happy" or "very happy" among 60 participants in that study) with both conventional and crossed IOL patterns; the spectacle independence rate was also impressive: only 1 patient among the 30 conventional IOL monovision group needed reading glasses "all the time"

and 3 patients among the 30 crossed IOL monovision group needed reading glasses "all the time." For distance-related activities, 86.6% in the conventional group "never or only occasionally need glasses" and 90% in the crossed IOL monovision group "never or only occasionally need glasses."

A study by Fawcett et al[55] with 32 adults who had post-LASIK/PRK monovision after more than 6 months of follow-up demonstrated a difference of stereoacuity in the two groups: low anisometropia (< 1.50 D) versus moderate anisometropia (1.50 D or more). Median stereoacuity values were 100 seconds of arc for patients with low anisometropia and 150 seconds of arc for patients with moderate anisometropia.

Our own 10-year IOL monovision review found complete spectacle freedom in 36.2% of a low anisometropic group (0.75–1.0 D, mean: 0.88 ± 0.12 D), 46.9% in a modest anisometropic group (1.01–1.50 D, mean: 1.31 ± 0.13D), and 40.9% in a high anisometropic group (> 1.50 D, mean: 1.93 ± 0.25 D), although there was no statistically significant difference among these results. Modest level anisometropia (mean, 1.31 D) had a higher rate of complete spectacle independence than either the low (mean, 0.88 D) or the high anisometropia group (mean, 1.93 D). That result was *not* expected because we previously assumed that a higher anisometropia level would have a higher rate of glasses freedom. In that study, the > 1.50 group had a higher rate of needing glasses for nighttime driving; this was probably the main reason why complete spectacle freedom was lower in the high anisometropia group (mean, 1.93 D) than the modest group (mean, 1.31 D). The rate of needing glasses all the time for nighttime driving in that study was 21.9% in the high group, 15.3% in the modest group, and 14.8% in the low group. There was no statistically significant difference in the trend *p*-value (0.438).

Monovision has some inevitable limitations. Once the near eye is –1.50 D or more, the intermediate vision, stereovision, and contrast will show a more noticeable negative impact. Ambati et al[21] noted that stereovision decreased greatly when the blur was more than 1.75 D. A study by Loshin et al[53] demonstrated that, up to a moderate anisometropic level of 1.50 D, monovision blur appeared to have a limited negative impact on high-frequency contrast sensitivity and binocular summation, but as add power increased, the whole frequency range was involved and binocular summation significantly decreased.

An experimental study was conducted by Schor et al[56] with different anisometropic levels at 1.25, 1.75, and 2.50 D in different luminance testing environments to mimic nighttime driving. The study revealed that interocular suppression of blur was greater with lower level anisometropia, which means better monovision function, which was less likely to produce asthenopia. Five binocularly normal participants in an experimental study by Simpson[57] suggested that anisometropic blur induces a central suppression scotoma in the defocused eye. The suppression scotoma was shown to increase in size as the degree of anisometropia increased.

Pardhan and Gilchrist[52] studied 10 young healthy participants aged 17 to 28 years with a + 0.50, + 1.00, + 1.50, + 2.00, + 2.50, + 3.00, or + 3.50 D defocusing lens placed over one eye to compare contrast sensitivity. That study demonstrated that the maximum contrast sensitivity was in the absence of any monocular defocusing, with full binocular summation, about 42% higher than the monocular value. Monovision up to 1.50 D would still show binocular summation, but the binocular summation disappeared when the monocular defocusing power reached 1.50 D. The study also showed a phenomenon called binocular inhibition, defined as a condition where binocular is lower than monocular sensitivity. Binocular inhibition did not seem to occur until the defocusing add reached 1.50 D. As the power approached + 2.50 D, the binocular inhibition reached its maximum level. As the power of the defocusing lens increased, the binocular sensitivity reverted back to the monocular level, indicating suppression of the defocused eye. Binocular inhibition was also noted objectively in a study done by Trick et al[58] in which 10 normal young participants were tested with visual evoked responses (VERs) with different levels of neutral density filters. In a typical binocular situation, both eyes view the same stimulus pattern and the amplitude of the binocular VER is approximately 1.4 times larger than the amplitude of either monocular response, but when the luminance difference between the two eyes was large enough, the amplitude of VER of both eyes became smaller than the amplitude of *either* monocular VER. These interesting studies remind us to consider the threshold or zone for our IOL monovision practice: which level of anisometropia would be most likely to give our patients the best balanced visual function?

Stereopsis and both photopic and mesopic sensitivity decreased as the add increased from 0.75 to 1.75 D in an experimental study of 82 simulated pseudophakic monovision patients by Hayashi et al.[51] The same study suggested 1.50 D anisometropia as the optimal refraction for IOL monovision based on the balance of vision for distance, intermediate and near, stereopsis, and contrast sensitivity.

With optical analysis, we can demonstrate the difference in the not-sharply-focused-zone (NSFZ) between modest monovision and full monovision. If OD is plano with 20/20 vision and OS has −1.50 D IOL monovision in a 60-year-old bilateral pseudophake, assuming a pseudophakic accommodating power average of 1.00 D, the length of the NSFZ is 33.3 cm, from 100 to 66.7 cm. However, if we give OS −2.50 D IOL monovision for the same patient, the NSFZ will be 60 cm, between 100 and 40 cm. (See the section "Optics and Neurophysiology of Pseudophakic Monovision" in Chapter 2 for details.)

Duke-Elder and Abrams claimed that each 0.25 D difference between the refraction of the two eyes causes 0.5% difference in size between the two retinal images and a difference of 5% is the limit which can usually be tolerated with ease.[59] They also mentioned that patients might experience discomfort when they have more than 2.00 D anisometropia due to an artificial heterophoria.

A Case Report

A female patient of F. Z. was 50 years old when she came to have a cataract evaluation in 2002. She had a posterior subcapsular cataract (PSC) in her left eye. Her left eye was dominant. Left eye cataract surgery was performed in January 2003 with a 20/20 uncorrected distance vision result. Her right eye, also with a PSC cataract, was operated on in May 2007. It was aimed at −2.15 D but ended up at −2.75 D. Manifest refraction did not show significant astigmatism. Vision of her right eye was 20/20 with −2.75 D. Overall, she has been happy without glasses or contact lens for most daily activities, especially for reading and her job as a dental hygienist. The only time she needs backup aid is for nighttime driving. She uses both glasses and contact lenses as single vision for distance as a backup, but she much prefers to wear a contact lens for her right eye for nighttime driving rather than use her backup glasses. It is likely that it is more comfortable for her to wear a contact lens for her right eye than to wear a pair of glasses for her right eye correction of −2.75 and left eye correction of plano due to the difference of aniseikonia. At 2.75 D, aniseikonia would be 6% with spectacles but only 0.5% with contact lenses. At her visit in

February 2017, a prescription for backup glasses was given: plano on top OU with + 1.50 bifocal OU because of her complaint of not being able to clearly see the dashboard when she was driving at nighttime with her contact lens in her right eye. She does not need to wear any glasses or contact lens during the daytime. Retrospectively, I wish I had aimed her right eye at –1.50 D only, since arm's length vision was the main need for her job. I predominantly used traditional full monovision at a level around 2.00 D in my early career years.

4.5.2 Full Monovision Still Has a Role to Meet Some Patients' Needs

The above discussion clearly demonstrates the negative effect of full monovision on stereopsis and contrast. From our own study, we also documented that full IOL monovision patients have a greater chance of needing glasses for nighttime driving. It will be interesting to find out the long-term impact on ocular muscle alignment in our full monovision patient population. Having said that, full monovision still has a role to meet some patients' needs, although we must be more cautious in our decision-making process.

A study in 2002 by Greenbaum[5] consisting of 140 IOL monovision patients (120 with visually significant cataract and 20 with clear lens exchange for high ametropia) demonstrated a 92% (129 patients) success rate. The subjective criterion for success was patient acceptance and satisfaction with IOL monovision at a 6-month or 1-year final interview. The objective criteria were uncorrected distance vision of 20/30 or better and uncorrected near vision J1 or better. In that study, the dominant eye was aimed to be emmetropic and the nondominant eye was targeted at –2.75. The spectacle dependence rate for distance was 5.8% and for near was 8.4%. There were no stereovision or contrast tests reported in the study.

In a prospective comparison study[2] in 2011 between IOL monovision and multifocal IOLs, we found that most near-full monovision patients did very well: 77% (17/22) never needed reading glasses; 81.8% (18/22) were "very happy" and "absolutely would recommend it to family members." In terms of overall patient satisfaction and significant visual complaints, the monofocal IOL monovision group did better than the multifocal IOL group. The average refractive power in the near vision eye in the monovision group was –1.92 D, with a median of 1.88 D.

A Case Report

A 65-year-old well-educated woman whose occupation involved doing payrolls presented in 2014 for cataract evaluation. She complained of decreased vision in both eyes, especially when driving. Her uncorrected distance vision was OD 20/200 and OS 20/100; uncorrected near vision was OD J1 and OS J1 +. Her corrected distance vision was OD 20/40 and OS 20/30. Preoperative refraction was OD –2.75D and OS –2.25D. Hole-in-card and camera tests showed that the right eye was dominant. Past ocular history and the cover and uncover test revealed no contraindication for IOL monovision. She had been wearing a contact lens for OD only for 15 years and her OS was her near eye without a contact lens. She wanted to keep her monovision. Her three main hobbies were cooking, biking, and shopping. The decision for her refractive goal was made based on these main hobbies: OD plano and OS –1.25 D. The right eye was done in June 2014 and left eye in July 2014. She came back 2 years later, with OD 20/20 plano and OS 20/20 –1.00 D sphere. Near vision without correction OD was J16 and OS J7. She wore + 1.50 D readers. She was not happy with the reading ability of her left eye. She wanted to know if she could get rid of the readers. "Make my left eye stronger so I do not have to wear readers." To make sure that full permanent monovision was what she really liked, a trial contact lens was offered. She preferred + 1.75 D over her left eye rather than + 1.50 D. Popular piggyback IOLs with 0.50 D increments, such as the Staar AQ5010, was not available anymore, so we had to choose either a + 2.00 D or + 3.00 D Alcon MA60MA 3 piece sulcus lens. A + 2.00 D lens would give a refractive outcome of around –2.25D and a + 3.00D lens would give an outcome between –2.75 D and – 3.00D. She strongly preferred + 3.00 D. "With the contact lens of + 1.75 and my –1.00 myopia, I can read very well, so near –3.00 will be just fine for me." (She was amazingly familiar with the optics.) Surgery was done in November 2016 (F. Z.'s second monovision-related piggyback IOL in 20 years). Postoperative uncorrected distance vision was OD 20/20, OS 20/400; corrected distance vision was OD plano 20/20, OS 20/20 with –2.75. Uncorrected near vision were OD J16 and OS J1 +. Stereopsis and contrast sensitivity tests showed significant decreases comparing full monovision with the piggyback with modest monovision prior to piggyback (▶ Table 4.1 and ▶ Table 4.2).

Table 4.1 Preoperative and postoperative stereopsis comparison

Stereopsis	
Pre-op	Post-op
4/9 circles 140 seconds of arc	2/9 circles 400 seconds of arc

Table 4.2 Preoperative and postoperative contrast sensitivity comparison

	Contrast sensitivity test results			
	Day		Night	
	Pre-op	Post-op	Pre-op	Post-op
RE	1.35	1.35	1.20	1.20
LE	1.35	1.05	1.35	1.05
BE	1.65	1.50	1.50	1.35

Despite the downside from full monovision of 2.75 D, she is very happy with her overall condition and does not have any complaints. However, when she was asked if she noted any other differences between prepiggyback and postpiggyback, she acknowledged that she has to use backup glasses more often for nighttime driving and also has to get closer to her computer. That situation fits what we discussed in the section "The Not-Sharply-Focused-Zone in Full Monovision" in Chapter 2.

4.5.3 A Customized Approach Is Preferred

Generally speaking, "one-size-fits-all" is not the best approach for IOL monovision refractive cataract surgery. The best approach is a customized plan to match each patient's daily life needs. It is more important to make the patient happy than to have a higher spectacle independence rate. If a retired patient loves outdoor activities and computer work, but does not do much small print reading and does not mind backup readers, then a modest monovision plan with the dominant eye at plano to –0.25 D and nondominant fellow eye at around –1.00 D to –1.25 D will be excellent for that patient. IOL mini-monovision did not seem to cause any problems in our practices as long as the patient understood the possible need and was willing to use backup readers for small print. If a patient requests to be glasses free for both far and near with reading as the priority goal, then aiming the nondominant eye at –1.50 to –2.00 D will be very appropriate. Full monovision will offer a chance of being completely glasses free for almost all daily activities except nighttime driving. These patients can be very happy with their visual function. The downside is that, as the anisometropia level increases, stereovision decreases, especially if the nondominant eye ends up more myopic due to biometry errors. Then the patient will be more likely to need glasses or contact lenses more than originally hoped to achieve comfortable bilateral vision.

A patient's job should also be an important factor to consider. For example, for a professional truck driver, the reasonable setting of dominant distance vision is at plano to –0.25 D and the reading eye at –0.75 D. With this plan, he will have great distance vision and reasonable arm's length vision to take care of his dashboard without glasses. If a dental hygienist requests to be glasses free for her work, but does not mind having backup glasses for far, then aiming the dominant eye at –1.00 D and the nondominant eye at –2.00 D will be more likely to make her happy without any glasses at the office while still having great near stereovision for her job.

It is worth mentioning that clinicians may often overvalue total spectacle freedom as the index of patient satisfaction when we practice IOL monovision. Customizing individual needs and making patients happy should be the priority.

4.5.4 Keep the Dominant Eye Plano or Slightly Myopic

Aiming the dominant eye between plano and –0.25 D seems to be a well-accepted practice. Targeting a very small amount of myopic defocus for the dominant distance eye, typically no more than –0.25 D is our personal preference, not only provides less chance to end up with a hyperopic result, which will need more ciliary muscle strength for accommodation, but also adds additional reading power to the distance eye. The literature has richly demonstrated good clinical results with a small amount of myopia for the dominant distance eye. A recent clinical experimental study by Naeser et al[60] in Denmark with 22 pseudophakic patients, average age 66 years and 8 weeks postoperative, suggested that –0.25 and –1.25 D pseudophakic monovision may be the optimal choice to provide spectacle independence for distance and intermediate vision and increased depth of focus with minimal negative compromise for binocular visual functions, such as stereovision, contrast, and monovision suppression.

4.5.5 Summary of Preferred Anisometropia Level for IOL Monovision

Mini-monovision works well for those patients who want to have good distance and intermediate vision without glasses. Anisometropia of 1.00 to 1.50 D should work well for the majority of patients with better binocular stereopsis and contrast, although they may have to use backup glasses for prolonged reading of small print. At this level, even in patients with strong ocular dominance, which is not always easy to pick up in our current preoperative testing, asthenopia is unlikely to occur. This level of anisometropia can be considered physiological, allowing fusion and binocular summation rather than suppression that may be necessary with higher levels of anisometropia. Traditional monovision with the near eye at −1.75 to −2.50 D typically can have a higher rate of reading glasses independence but may have a more noticeable impact on stereopsis and contrast sensitivity. It is advisable to consult each individual patient for his/her personal preferences and visual needs in a customized approach. For novice clinicians, it will be better to start with mini- or modest monovision.

4.6 Which Eye for Distance and Which Eye for Near?

For this topic, the following factors should be considered:

- Sighting dominance test.
- Distance vision and the cataract density of each eye.
- Refractive status of each eye.
- History of monovision.
- Longstanding weaker eye.
- Ocular comorbidity.
- Crossed IOL monovision.

4.6.1 Sighting Dominance Test

Correcting the dominant eye for distance and the nondominant eye for near is the conventional monovision approach. There is abundant evidence that this conventional approach typically yields a high level of satisfying results for vision and spectacle independence,[2,3,5,7,19,39,40,61] with the assumption that it is easier for the dominant eye to suppress the blur induced in the nondominant eye during distance viewing.[17,20] There is also evidence to suggest that crossed monovision works

well,[4,12] but crossed monovision may have a higher chance of causing fixation switch diplopia if some potential contraindications, such as monofixation syndrome, borderline phoria, and amblyopia, which may be asymptomatic, are not excluded in candidates.[55,62,63,64] (See details in the section "Potential Contraindications and Concerns for Pseudophakic Monovision" later in the chapter.) Except for specific conditions discussed later, choosing the dominant eye with the hole-in-card test for distance is recommended.

4.6.2 Distance Vision and the Density of the Cataract of Each Eye

There is no fixed pattern of vision and sighting dominance,[16,28] but we usually see that better distance vision is with the sighting dominant eye. The denser cataract eye typically causes worse preoperative vision. It is not hard to make a decision if the vision and lens density match the sighting dominance hole-in-card test; but if they do not match, personally I (FZ) would still make the decision to follow the hole-in-card test.

4.6.3 Refractive Status

The less myopic eye is often preferred for distance and the more myopic eye for near in the preoperative stage. This is similar in hyperopia, but it seems to be more variable. The eye with no astigmatism or less astigmatism is often the better seeing eye in the preoperative stage. It is reasonable to keep the same pattern for postoperative choices.

4.6.4 History of Monovision

If a patient has a history of monovision with good results and no complaints, or is currently using monovision, especially for a long duration, no matter whether due to natural monovision, contact lenses, laser vision correction, refractive status change, or cataract formation, stick to the same pattern, regardless of the dominant eye test. It does not seem to matter if the monovision is conventional or crossed from the dominance point of view. If you turn around and change the pattern, it might cause a situation similar to forcing a right-handed person to write with the left hand.

A Case Report

This was my (F.Z.) first piggyback IOL experience with reversing monovision. A lady in her 70 s with a history of contact lens monovision for about 10 years was using her OS only for near. "Never had any problem with monovision." She had no contact lens for the last few years due to "dry eye." She wanted cataract surgery and to keep monovision. She had no contraindications for IOL monovision by history and by ocular examination including cover and uncover test.

Her OD vision was worse than OS at presentation due to a denser cataract and likely some myopic shift in OD. OS was her dominant eye with the hole-in-card test at presentation.

The decision was to choose the dominant eye OS for far and the nondominant eye OD for near based on the hole-in-card test. Surgery was uneventful in both eyes and there was no need to correct astigmatism in either eye. Postoperative vision was good OD for near and OS for far without correction. After she recovered from a long hospitalization for her chronic obstructive pulmonary disease (COPD), she came back to me complaining that "Something is not right. I do not feel comfortable when I am reading." Ocular examination was unremarkable.

A pair of customized reading glasses was prescribed to yield good reading vision for OS. The patient did not have any ocular complaint at the follow-up visit except that she did not like the reading glasses "They hurt my ears because of my O2 line on my ears." She refused to use contact lenses again. She took the option of a piggyback IOL to reverse OS for reading and OD for distance. She was basically wheelchair bound from her COPD and reading was her main hobby, so a piggyback IOL was first done in her OS for reading.

She remained complaint free after OS reversal for reading, so the plan to reverse OD for far was cancelled. She had a long history of contact lens monovision, OS for near prior to her cataract formation. Her OD was her real motor sighting dominant eye. Her OS became the dominant eye when OD became more myopic with denser cataract formation and worse vision. As we know, ocular dominance can change when vision changes and refractive status changes.

The take-home message from this case is that it is a good idea to keep the monovision pattern if the patient was doing well in the past with contact lens–induced or laser vision correction–induced monovision. A sighting dominance test such as the hole-in-card can be plastic as the vision changes and/or as the refractive status changes.

4.6.5 Longstanding Weaker Eye

It is advisable for IOL monovision practice to remember to always ask this question to any prospective patient: Can you recall if you have one eye which is always weaker than the other eye? If yes, pay close attention to the cover and uncover test, do a stereopsis test with the best manifest correction, and then include the reading add; do a W4D test and 4-diopter prism base-out test to make sure that that patient does not have amblyopia, or a monofixation syndrome. (See the section "Potential Contraindications and Concerns for Pseudophakic Monovision" regarding how to detect subtle contraindications.) If no contraindication is found, personally I (FZ) would then avoid choosing that weaker eye for the distance eye. The "weaker" eye could be just due to greater astigmatism, or a more myopic or hyperopic refractive status. It is our anecdotal experience that amblyopia patients do not do well with IOL monovision because the healthy eye is so dominant that the image from the weak eye will not be clear due to the lack of enough interocular suppression of the healthy eye. Longstanding unilateral traumatic dense cataracts probably should be avoided for the dominant distance eye. Those patients may have compromised fusion function and therefore may have postoperative double vision to start with, especially if the vision loss is longer than 2 years or if the eye already has a motor deviation. (See the section "Potential Contraindications and Concerns for Pseudophakic Monovision.")

4.6.6 Ocular Comorbidity

Patients with severe ocular comorbidities are not good candidates for IOL monovision: severe maculopathy due to age-related wet macular degeneration, severe diabetic retinopathy, severe peripheral field loss in advanced glaucoma, or hemianopia after cerebral stroke, just to name a few. However, occasionally patients are very motivated to get as much spectacle independence as possible; in those situations, it is quite reasonable to consider IOL monovision if the ocular comorbidities are not severe and if the patient understands the limitations and the likelihood of needing glasses in the future. The eye with more central vision compromise, as in macular pathology, or central fixation involvement in glaucomatous field damage is usually wise to avoid for the dominant distance eye. Some case reports are given in Chapter 5 "Ocular Comorbidity and Pseudophakic Monovision."

4.6.7 Crossed IOL Monovision

We do sometimes run into situations where crossed IOL monovision is needed, choosing the dominant eye for near and the nondominant eye for far. For example, if you operate on the nondominant eye first, aiming for −1.0 D, but it ends up as −0.25 D with good uncorrected distance vision, then you may need to choose the dominant eye for near as crossed monovision or abandon the original monovision plan. Or, sometimes a patient may change his or her mind after the first eye was done and then want to have the unoperated eye cover whatever the first eye was not able to see clearly without glasses. Generally speaking, crossed IOL monovision works well in most patients if contraindications are avoided and if anisometropia is at a mini or modest level.[4,12] With this knowledge and experience, clinicians often can double their chance to achieve glasses independence for their patients. Generally speaking, we still recommend the conventional monovision pattern if possible, since crossed monovision may have a higher chance of causing fixation switch diplopia, or disturbing borderline balanced ocular alignment, if we fail to avoid potential contraindications, such as monofixation syndrome, borderline phoria, mild amblyopia, or longstanding unilateral dense cataract.[55,62,63,64] More details are discussed in the contraindication section. See the section "Potential Contraindications and Concerns for Pseudophakic Monovision."

4.6.8 Summary of IOL Monovision Types

Conventional IOL monovision is still the preferred pattern, although crossed IOL monovision also works well as long as the anisometropia level is modest and contraindications are avoided.[4,12] If a patient has a history of monovision and doing well without problems, keep the same pattern regardless of the dominant eye test.

4.7 Which Eye to Operate upon First?

The following factors are usually considered, but they can vary depending on each individual patient's condition.

4.7.1 Usually, the Worse Vision Eye Should Be Done First to Improve Vision

Most patients prefer this pattern.

4.7.2 If Cataract Density and Vision Are About Equal, Operate on the Nondominant Eye First

This will give some chance for adjustment to the dominant eye in case the refractive status is not perfectly reached in the first operated eye.[65] Generally speaking, to be able to give the dominant eye good distance vision without glasses is more important than correcting the nondominant eye for near.

4.7.3 If Both Eyes Are Highly Myopic, Operate on the More Myopic Eye First

This will leave a lesser degree of anisometropia between the two eyes after the first eye operation while waiting for the second eye surgery—for example, if the preoperative refraction is OD −4.00 D and OS −6.00 D and if OD is the dominant eye and the plan is to aim for plano OD and −1.50 D OS. If we operate on OD first, the patient will have to deal with 6.00 D anisometropia before the second eye operation. If we operate OS first aiming at −1.50 D, the patient will be left with 2.50 D anisometropia to deal with in the period of waiting for the second eye surgery. The advantage of operating the higher refractive eye in high hyperopia is not as great as it is in high myopia—for example, if the OD is + 4.00 D and OS + 6.00 D with OD as dominant eye. If we operate OS first aiming at −1.50 D, it will leave 5.50 D anisometropia. If we operate OD first aiming plano, it will leave 6.00 D anisometropia between the two eye operations. The waiting period between the two eyes in our practice (F. Z.) is typically longer than 4 weeks, which can be a significant challenge for the patient to handle if the induced anisometropia level is high in the interval between the two operations, especially if the patient is still working.

4.7.4 Focus on the Priority Goal

I have noted that this strategy can be quite helpful for those patients with very demanding personalities, although this is my (FZ) personal recommendation.

Missing the refractive target can occur, although it is rare with the advanced preoperative biometry and intraoperative aberration measurement tools now available. To regain the planned target, we can do LASIK or PRK, IOL exchange, or insert a piggyback IOL, but if we cannot make the patient happy the first time, the value from the second surgery to correct the mistake in the first eye will be discounted. One of the poorly recognized and underused strategies is to focus on the priority goal. Have your patient tell you the priority goal at the preoperative consultation. Have each prospective IOL monovision patient make a list of three common things he or she does most, which they would prefer to do without glasses. The first in the list should be the number one priority among the three. Make an effort to ensure that this priority is met. If a patient has a priority to be glasses free for far, then do the dominant eye first aiming for plano to –0.25D. If the priority is for reading, do the nondominant eye first aiming for –1.25 to –1.50 D. The surgeon will have two chances to achieve one priority goal, although for overwhelmingly most conditions, we can get what we plan from the first eye operation.

For example, if the priority is for distance, you do the dominant eye first. If the first eye did not get what you planned, say –0.50 D with UCDV 20/30 and UCNV 20/40. At this point, spend extra time with the patient to discuss what to do for the second eye with the following questions:

- Is the patient happy? If yes, then with what? Happy with distance or with near?
- Make sure to ask the patient if he or she is happy with the operated eye function alone. That means, the evaluation was done monocularly, not binocularly. If the unoperated eye is –2.00 with 3 + NS cataract and if we just ask the patient "Can you read well without glasses?" The answer may be "Yes, I have no problem to read without glasses." However, the reality is that it could be due to the then unoperated eye reading power, not from the operated eye.
- If the patient is indeed happy with the original plan to cover distance vision without glasses, then you can keep the original plan to make the second eye the near eye.
- If the patient is not happy with the priority goal for distance, but ok with the near vision from the operated eye, then you can aim the second eye for plano as crossed IOL monovision. This focus on the priority goal gives you a second chance to make the patient happy.
- If the patient is not happy for distance nor near with the operated eye, the discussion at this

point should be focused on with which eye to compromise. Usually, the patient favors their priority; that means, you will have another chance to reach the priority goal.

Let us take a look at another example. If the priority is to read without spectacles and you operate on the nondominant eye first, aiming at –1.50 D but it ends up at –0.75 D with UCDV 20/30 and UCNV 20/30, what should you do? If the patient is happy with the near vision, then keep your original plan to aim the second eye for plano. If the patient is not happy with the reading vision, then aim the second eye for –1.75 to –2.00 D.

The merits of focusing on the priority are twofold: it provides the surgeon two chances to reach the number one goal and it provides a mental cushion for the patient. Discussion of this process with the patient preoperatively alone prepares the patient for a realistic outcome. Make the patient understand that variation does occur, although it is rare. By knowing that crossed IOL monovision works as well as conventional IOL monovision as a group when anisometropia is kept at a modest level and contraindications are avoided, we can feel very comfortable using this modality to deal with some unexpected outcomes. Also, by learning that the refraction is off-target from the first operated eye, we typically can do better for the second eye by fine-tuning the IOL power calculation.[65] With modern biometry and intraoperative aberrometry, the chance of hitting the refractive target is typically very high with a single attempt, but the strategy of focusing on the priority offers extra backup for these demanding patients. I (FZ) have kept patients with very demanding personalities out of IOL monovision for a long time, but not over the last 4 to 5 years. I (FZ) have not run into any issue since we have adapted this "focus on the priority goal" strategy in the last 4 to 5 years among those demanding personality patients.

4.7.5 Summary: Which Eye to Operate First?

Generally speaking, we should operate on the eye with the denser cataract or worst vision or the nondominant eye first. For demanding personality patients, focusing on the priority goal will give the surgeon two chances to reach the priority refractive target. If the priority is for far vision, operate on the distance eye first; if the priority is for near vision, then operate on the near eye first.

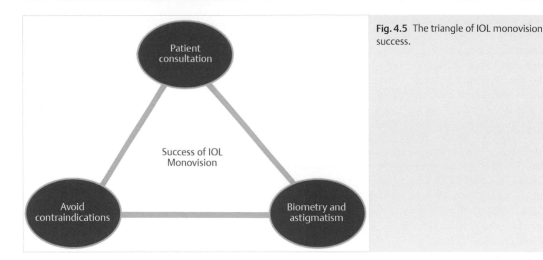

Fig. 4.5 The triangle of IOL monovision success.

4.8 Potential Contraindications and Concerns for Pseudophakic Monovision

Avoiding contraindications is one of the three key factors to achieve IOL monovision success (▶ Fig. 4.5). That also seems to be one of the main reasons why some surgeons are reluctant to initiate intentional IOL monovision, since they do not know what should be avoided.

4.8.1 Ocular Contraindications and Concerns

Tropia and Significant Phoria

Generally speaking, a patient with a noticeable tropia does not have fusion function and should be avoided for pseudophakic monovision. There are some rare exceptions where intentional monovision to correct longstanding stable diplopia may be reasonable (see Chapter 5, section "Monovision to Correct Diplopia").

Mild phoria should be acceptable for monovision, but it is advisable not to offer IOL monovision to patients who have more than 10 D of exophoria.[40] Patients with 12 or more esophoria with Maddox Rod were not considered for IOL monovision by McDonald and Rotramel.[66] A retrospective study consisting of 60 IOL monovision patients with 5-year postoperative data by Ito et al[40] noted a significant difference in small-angle exophoria (10 prism diopter or less) versus moderate exophoria (more than 10 prism diopter). Although none of the patients in both groups had developed permanent exotropia for distance fixation in the 5-year study duration, in the moderate exophoria group 60.5% developed intermittent exotropia. More patients failed the W4D test in the moderate exophoria group. The authors recommended that for those patients who have moderate angle exophoria, pseudophakic monovision application should be cautiously considered.

For any significant phoria patient, we recommend a full history and careful tests to rule out amblyopia and monofixation syndrome using the near Titmus stereo, 4-diopter prism base-out and W4D tests. Significant phoria patients with suboptimal fusion ability may not have enough capacity to handle the extra load of anisometropia with a risk of developing a manifest deviation.

Preexisting Significant Anisometropia

History of preexisting anisometropia prior to cataract formation is another thing to look at carefully before we decide to offer IOL monovision. These patients can either be great candidates for IOL monovision due to their natural monovision or have hidden monofixation syndrome and amblyopia. It is not rare to see some patients with 1.00 to 2.00 D of anisometropia but without any sign of amblyopia or monofixation. These can be excellent candidates for IOL monovision. Keeping the same pattern for far and near is recommended. On the flip side, in young children, > 1.50 D of hyperopic anisometropia or > 3.00 D of myopic anisometropia has significant potential to cause amblyopia.[67]

Parks stated that in young children, 1.50 D aniso-metropia increases the risk of monofixation to about 50% and 2.00 D almost 100%.[67] Thus, high preexisting anisometropia should be a red flag for the clinician; it deserves further exploration for both detailed past ocular history and testing.

History of Strabismus

Pollard et al[49] reported a study of 12 patients who had the onset of strabismus or recurrence of stra-bismus after obtaining monovision via contact lenses, LASIK, and cataract surgery with PCIOLs. Most of them were aged 40 to 50. Three of them had IOL monovision and the rest had contact lens-, LASIK-, or RK-induced monovision. Seven regained fusion by doing away with monovision and five required surgery to reestablish motor or sensory control. All of the surgery patients obtained excel-lent alignment but one did not regain sensory fusion. The authors of the study reached the follow-ing cautious conclusion: "Monovision is successful for the far majority of patients who try it. However, in patients with a previous history of strabismus or those with significant phoria, caution should be used in recommending monovision."

Kushner[62] reported 16 cases of acquired diplopia in those who had a history of strabismus or amblyopia since childhood. Six out of 16 were due to monovision correction.

We would not recommend IOL monovision to any patients if they had a history of prism usage, double vision, strabismus, or extraocular muscle surgery, or if they currently have a tropia or signif-icant phoria at the decision-making visit prior to cataract surgery, unless you plan to use the mono-vision modality to purposefully correct preexisting diplopia (see further discussion in the section "Monovision To Correct Diplopia" in Chapter 5). Routinely offering IOL monovision to any cataract patient without a good history and a careful cover and uncover test can be risky. It is not rare for some clinicians to routinely offer IOL monovision to cataract patients without any detailed history or preoperative screening tests.

Longstanding Unilateral Dense Cataract

For unilateral longstanding dense cataract, espe-cially traumatic cataract, even if the eyes do not seem to have strabismus, they may already have compromised central fusion. If they do have some strabismus, of course, we should not offer any IOL monovision, especially crossed IOL monovision. It can be difficult or impossible to accurately evaluate ocular alignment if the strabismus is small in those longstanding unilateral cataract patients due to poor vision and poor fixation from the dense cata-ract. For those patients, warning of the possibility of postoperative diplopia is warranted, even if the cataract is not traumatic and even if the eyes appear to be straight. If preoperative strabismus is noted on examination due to the longstanding uni-lateral cataract, even if the trauma happened dur-ing adulthood, there is a good chance that such a patient will have diplopia after the surgery.[68,69,70] This is possibly due to fusion disruption. Pratt-Johnson and Tillson[69] reported 24 cases of unilat-eral longstanding traumatic cataract from 1984 to 1988. All of these 24 cases had unilateral traumatic cataracts and had intractable diplopia after their vision was restored with IOLs or contact lenses to 20/40 vision or better. None of these 24 cases had a known history of interrupted binocular function prior to their trauma and the average age at the trauma was 18 years old (from 6 to 39). There was no central nervous system trauma associated with the ocular trauma. The study noted that the risk of diplopia increased if the interval from cataract for-mation to vision restoration reached 2.5 years or longer. The authors also noted that these patients typically had secondary strabismus in the injured eye, 1 year or longer after the injury. Occluding the eye might be the only way to deal with this kind of intractable diplopia, per that study.[69]

How to approach a longstanding unilateral dense cataract? I (FZ) personally recommend no IOL mono-vision until the first eye surgery has been done and postoperative binocular function is reassessed. It is reasonable to correct the affected eye aiming for it to be slightly more myopic than the fellow normal or less dense cataract eye. If postoperative tests show good stereovision and fusion, then consider the IOL monovision option at the time of the fellow eye sur-gery if the patient requires glasses independence.

Monofixation Syndrome

Monofixation syndrome is a loss of bifixation or foveal fusion resulting in the manifestation of a fac-ultative absolute scotoma in the fovea of the nonfix-ating eye.[55,63,71] The absence of foveal fusion that characterizes monofixation syndrome can occur in strabismic and orthotropic eyes.[63,71] Because of the fact that some monofixation patients are orthophoric, especially those with primary mono-fixation syndrome, trying to avoid any tropia and > 8 to 10 D phoria as the recommendation for IOL monovision is not safe enough, because one-third of monofixation patients show orthophoria with the cover and uncover test.[63] They maintain good peripheral fusion. Two-thirds of monofixation syndrome patients were noted to have amblyopia, but one-third were not amblyopic and alternated their fixation, simultaneously transferring the mac-ular scotoma from eye to eye.[67]

Preoperative examination with a stereopsis test, 4-D base-out prism test, and/or W4D fusion at a distance of 6 m is helpful to make the diagnosis, although it may not be reliable if the cataract is dense and vision is very poor. Of note, normal fusion with the W4D test at near does not rule out monofixation because normal peripheral fusion may still be maintained.[63] Since most of the scoto-mas of monofixating patients are approximately 3 degrees, most, if not all, monofixation syndrome patients can fuse at 13 inches with the W4D test but are unable to fuse at a distance of 20 feet.[63] If eccentric fixation is present in one eye, the cover and uncover test may not reveal any shift. One routinely asked question can be helpful: Are you aware of one eye always being weaker than the other eye for your whole life? If the answer is yes, then we should be careful about the decision to offer IOL monovision, although answering "yes" to that question does not necessarily mean that pa-tient is a monofixater. It can be due to refractive errors too. If the patient answers "no," it does not mean there is no problem, since the patient may not be aware of some mild conditions. The chal-lenge is that monofixation syndrome patients are often asymptomatic. Their eyes can be straight or nearly straight, with average fusional vergence amplitudes as bifixaters and appreciation of gross stereopsis and do not get worse as they age.[63]

Monofixation syndrome can be primary without any noticeable etiology, or secondary to small-angle strabismus, anisometropia, or a monocular macular lesion. Monofixation syndrome patients can become diplopic following mistakes in pre-scription of glasses, contact lenses, or IOLs. It can also develop after LASIK.[72]

The diagnosis of monofixation syndrome becomes clinically important when a clinician misses the diagnosis and chooses the nonfixating eye for distance. Fixation switch diplopia can occur as a consequence. Even conventional monovision will have a risk of breaking down the balance of

stable asymptomatic monofixation syndrome due to monovision-induced anisometropia.

A Case Report

A 60-year-old female executive had a preoperative history of hyperopia.[73] She had refractive lens exchange OD using a Restor 3D multifocal lens with an LRI, yielding 20/25 distance vision without correction, J8 at near without correction, and J3 with correction for OD. OS refracted with + 3.50 D, giving 20/20 acuity. There was no high-order aber-ration on iTrace with perfect optics OU. Two months postoperatively, she was not happy, and came for a second opinion. Recalled history: she had a patch over her left eye during childhood. A 4-D base-out prism test (4ΔBO) supported the diagnosis of monofixation of OS. The long duration of a weaker OD, now the fixating eye, was most likely the reason she was not happy. We believe that if the OS was corrected with a monofocal IOL at plano with 20/20 or better vision without cor-rection, the patient might be doing well. No fol-low-up information was available due to the nature of the consultation.

Fixation Switch Diplopia

Kushner[62] reported 16 cases of acquired diplopia as "fixation switch diplopia" in patients who had a his-tory of strabismus or amblyopia since childhood. Six out of 16 developed diplopia due to monovision correction because the nonfixating eye was made the fixating eye. In all 16 patients, symptoms were completely eliminated when optical correction was prescribed that restored the preferred eye for fixa-tion. In this nonalternating strabismus situation, with or without amblyopia, these patients may experience diplopia if they fixate with the eye that is not preferred. This has been referred to as "fixation switch diplopia."[62,64,68,74,75] It has been speculated that because the suppression that accompanies strabismus is facultative, suppression may not be present in the usually dominant eye when the nondominant eye is fixing.[75]

Boyd et al[64] reported a group of 24 patients with fixation switch diplopia who had spontaneous intermittent diplopia. All of these 24 patients had the following features: when they were asked to demonstrate the production of diplopia, each pa-tient fixed with the nonpreferred eye and no sup-pression was present in the preferred eye; when fixing with the preferred eye, suppression could be demonstrated in the nonpreferred eye and the diplopia disappeared. They were all able to alternate fixation, but not able to alternate suppression. That means that there was no alternate suppression present in these patients. Each of the 24 patients also had the squint onset before age 7 years and the preferred eye had better vision than the nonpreferred eye with vision of 20/20 or better in the good eye in all 24 cases.

Richards[74] reported 13 cases of patients with anisometropia who became diplopic when the previously less hyperopic fixating eye became myopic and the fixation switched to the previously nonfixating eye. Treatment with optical prescriptions or surgical correction of ocular alignment when necessary was quite successful for these patients, allowing a switch of fixation back to the originally fixating eye.[74]

A Case Report (Personal Communication with Lisa B. Arbisser, MD)[76]

A 69-year-old man was seen in August 2008 with a history of traumatic cataract in his left eye at age 10. He had no history of EOM surgery or diplopia. General health was unremarkable. Vision in the left eye was CF at 4 feet without correction, and 20/200 with –4.00 D. The right eye was dominant, also with a –4.00 D refraction. Preoperative examination revealed a mild cataract in the right eye with an epiretinal membrane. A decision was made to do cataract surgery on the left eye. Surgery was uneventful with a 15.50 D SN60WF IOL, and postoperative vision was 20/20 without correction. The patient also wanted right eye cataract surgery. Given that the preoperative refraction was –4.00 myopic, the decision was made to create monovision with the right eye aiming at –1.50 D. Surgery went well with an SN60WF 14.50 D IOL in the capsular bag. The patient was unhappy postoperatively despite achieving the aim of left eye 20/20 plano and right eye 20/25 with –1.50 D. He was not willing to wear glasses or contact lens, so a piggyback IOL was inserted in the right eye. A Starr AQ –2 D sulcus piggyback IOL placed 8 months after the original surgery resulted in 20/25 vision with plano, but pigment dispersion plus a steroid response caused ocular hypertension and secondary glaucoma. The piggyback IOL was removed and IOL exchanged 2 months later, using an MN60AC 11.50D IOL in the sulcus with optic capture with a result of plano, but CME and ERM with metamorphopsia ensued. A pars plana vitrectomy and membrane peeling was performed 6 months later with a result of 20/20 and plano OD. After that, it was first noticed he had 1 to 2 prism diopters of left hyperphoria, but the patient declined wearing glasses and seems to be doing well.

Why was that patient not happy after a successful surgery result of 20/20 and plano in the left eye and 20/25 with –1.50 D in the right eye? The assumption is that he had a strongly dominant right eye considering that he had trauma in his left eye at age 10 and the left eye had poor vision since then for 59 years. Now, the left eye was corrected to 20/20 with plano to function as the dominant eye and 20/25 with –1.5 D for the right eye to function for near vision. It is advisable to avoid choosing a long-term suppressed eye or amblyopic eye for distance vision eye if monovision is to be considered. One argument could be that it was caused by his 1 to 2 prism diopters of left hyperphoria, first noticed after all the surgeries were over, but still the patient seemed to be able to tolerate that misalignment well without any prism correction.

Amblyopia

In amblyopia, where strong ocular dominance is known to exist, patients tend to suppress information originating from the nondominant eye regardless of its clarity. These patients are not good candidates for monovision. It does not necessarily make the amblyopic eye worse, but from a spectacle independence point of view, it does not work well. In cases of borderline phoria, the extra anisometropic load from monovision can worsen the preexisting balance and may even lead to a manifest deviation.

A Case Report

A 61-year-old man with hyperopia OU and a history of amblyopia OD came for clear lens extraction with a strong desire not to wear glasses for far or near. He had no history of EOM surgery, prism use, or double vision. Preoperative refraction was OD + 5.75 + 0.25 × 039 giving 20/40 and OS + 6.00 sphere giving 20/20 acuity. Dominant eye tests noted OS as dominant with the hole-in-card and camera tests. Ocular exam was normal except for a trace epiretinal membrane in OD, but OCT was unremarkable. The W4D test at near showed four dots: two green and two yellow (not reported as red). W4D test at distance showed two dots: one green and one yellow. Cover and uncover test at distance with glasses: 4 prism diopter esophoria in primary gaze, left gaze, and right gaze, head tilt to right and to left. Monovision was planned with OD aimed at −1.00 and OS plano. Surgery was uneventful OU. Three months later, distance vision uncorrected was OD 20/50, OS 20/20, near vision uncorrected OD J5 and OS J3. Corrected distance vision OD −1.25 + 0.50 × 027 20/25 and OS plano 20/20. He stated that he did not need glasses for far, but needed glasses for arm's length such as using a computer and for all near work. For convenience, he wore glasses all the time. The fact that the anisometropia was low might also have played some role for his nonoptimal near vision, but uncorrected near vision was J5 OD, which was worse than his J3 OS. Uncorrected near vision was expected to be better in OD than OS if he did not have amblyopia in OD. At his 1-year postoperative visit, his ocular condition was the same. Monovision just did not work out well for this gentleman for his intermediate vision and his near vision. Fortunately, his cover and uncover test was the same with no deterioration at 1-year follow-up.

How to Detect Subtle Contraindications

As mentioned earlier in the monofixation section, some monofixation syndrome patients can have normal ocular alignment and no amblyopia. This can be a challenge for cataract surgeons. A detailed history and examination usually can detect these subtle contraindications.

Past Ocular History

A complete history is by far the most important part of the screening, though the physical examination can be limited due to the presence of the cataract. In our IOL monovision workup sheet, these questions are listed as musts to ask: Do you recall if you have one eye which is always weaker than the fellow eye for your whole life? Have you had any history of patching your eye when you were a child? Have you ever used a prism? Have you ever had double vision? If the history is positive, no monovision is offered in most situations. If it is suspicious, then a very through eye examination should not be neglected.

Examinations and Ocular Tests

Besides routine cover and uncover tests for every IOL monovision patient, the following three tests

are helpful for suspicious IOL monovision candidates:

Near Stereopsis with the Patient's Own Glasses or New Manifest Free Lenses

The Titmus test (Stereo Optical Co., Inc., Chicago, IL) is what we use. Great stereopsis suggests a low likelihood of past EOM problems, although a subnormal result could also be due to dense cataract or other ocular pathology.

Worth 4 Dot Tests with the Patient's Own Glasses or New Manifest Free Lenses

A normal distance W4D test suggests good fusion. A normal near W4D test does not rule out monofixation or mild amblyopia. An abnormal W4D test can also be due to dense cataract and/or other ocular comorbidity.

4 Diopter Base-Out Prism Test

The 4-D base-out prism test is performed primarily to document the presence of a small facultative scotoma in a patient with monofixation syndrome and no manifest deviation. In this test, a 4Δ base-out prism is quickly placed before one eye and then the other during binocular viewing, and motor responses are observed. Patients with bifixation usually show a version (bilateral) movement away from the eye covered by the prism followed by a unilateral fusional convergence movement of the eye not behind the prism. For example, if the prism is quickly placed in front of OD, then both eyes will show a quick movement to the left followed with convergence OS to resume fusion. If the prism is quickly placed in front of OS, both eyes will show a quick movement to the right side of the patient and then followed with OD convergence to resume fusion. In monofixation syndrome, when the prism is quickly placed in front of the fixating eye, it will cause both eyes to have a version movement away from the fixating eye, but no follow-up convergence from the nonfixating eye due to its central scotoma. If the base-out prism is quickly placed in front of the nonfixating eye (often mild amblyopic eye), no movement is seen from either eye.

There are some limitations to this 4-D base-out prism test.[77] An occasional patient with bifixation recognizes diplopia when the prism is placed before an eye but makes no convergence movement to correct for it. Patients with monofixation syndrome may switch fixation each time the prism is inserted and show no movement, regardless of which eye is tested. Even in normal bifixation patients, the bilateral version movement may not always be visible, especially in elderly cataract patients. The unilateral convergence from the eye which is not behind the prism can be a slow motion and not easily observable. In dense cataract with very poor vision, this test is almost impossible.

A Case Report

A 69-year-old female patient referred from an ophthalmologist for cataract evaluation and IOL monovision desired as much spectacle independence as possible. Her right eye vision had decreased more than her left eye over the last few years. "I happen to notice that I am using my right eye for near and left for far. Traffic signs, especially nighttime driving is very difficult for me now." She preferred to keep her "monovision" if it was not going to cause more problems. She recalled that she had a patch for her left eye when she was age 6 but her right eye vision was always as good as her left eye for her "whole life." The old records from her previous ophthalmologist noted corrected distance vision of 20/20 in each eye: OD $+1.00+0.50\times150$ and OS $+1.25+0.25\times015$. She never had double vision or prism use. At presentation, her vision OD was 20/50 with -2.50 and OS 20/25 with $-0.25+0.25\times005$. Her OD had $3+$ nuclear sclerosis (NS) and OS 2 to $3+$ NS cataract. OS was her dominant eye with the hole-in-card and camera tests. She had 4 PD exophoria in primary gaze, right gaze, left gaze, and on head tilt to the right and left. On the W4D test (red for her right eye and green for her left eye) at far, she was able to see only two green dots; at near she was normal, two green and two red. Stereo at near was 3/9. Four-diopter base-out prism placed in front of OS induced visible version movement away from the left to the right in each eye, but no following convergence movement by her OD. When it was placed in front of OD, neither eye showed any visible eye movement. Thus, the diagnoses were clear at that time: (1) cataract OU with significant NS and myopia shift in OD appears to be natural monovision, but her old note did not show this level of anisometropia; (2) amblyopia OD, very mild with patching history; (3) monofixation syndrome, OS is the fixating eye. The decision was to aim OD for -0.50 and OS for plano. (She had a strong desire to have reasonable vision for her cell phone without looking for readers.) OD surgery went well. She was doing well after her OD surgery. Her vision in her OD at 3-week follow-up was 20/20 with -0.50 D. She was very happy with her computer and cell phone vision without glasses. She preferred no surgery for her OS yet due to her busy working schedule. If we had missed these diagnoses and kept her prior full monovision, she may have developed a deteriorating phoria, possibly becoming a manifest tropia; and full monovision may not have worked well due to the strong dominance of her OS. She might have ended up needing glasses all of the time. If we operated on the worse eye (OD) first aiming for plano and then her dominant OS for near, she would likely have had a fixation switch issue with intolerable asthenopia.

4.8.2 Nonoptical or EOM-Related Severe Ocular Comorbidities

Severe ocular comorbidities can cause extensive damage, limiting the possibilities for IOL monovision: hemianopic field defect from stroke, constricted field from advanced glaucoma, advanced diabetic retinopathy, wet ARMD, etc. Generally, these patients should not be considered as candidates at all. Most patients with mild, and even some moderate ocular comorbidity, can actually do well with IOL monovision (see Chapter 5, Ocular Comorbitidies and Pseudophakic Monovision).

4.8.3 Systemic Contraindications and Concerns

Parkinson's Disease

Patients with some systemic situations, such as degenerative central nervous system diseases, where muscular function is compromised, should not be candidates for IOL monovision. Parkinson's disease is a typical example. Early in the course of the disease, the most obvious symptoms are movement related. All three fundamental types of eye movements can be involved: saccadic, pursuit, and vergence. In Parkinson's disease, the saccades tend to be slow. Some people with Parkinson's disease require a blink to change their saccadic position (Wilson's sign). This makes it difficult to fixate on changing targets in the environment and to read. When pursuit movements become decreased, this can produce jerky or cogwheel slow eye movements. The inadequacy or slowness of accommodation can result in eyestrain, vision fluctuation, headaches, and double vision when working on near tasks. Convergence insufficiency and ocular motor function have been demonstrated to be much worse than in an age matched control group.[78]

Graves' Eye Disease (GED)

GED, also known as thyroid eye disease, should not be considered for IOL monovision either. In this autoimmune condition, the body's immune system attacks extraocular muscles and orbital connective tissues. GED may occur in patients who already know they have thyroid disease, but sometimes it is the first problem that brings the patient to the doctor's office. The major problems of GED from an IOL monovision perspective are the tight orbit and eyelids, and the swelling of extraocular muscles, any of which may affect focusing and fusion and cause double vision.

Myasthenia Gravis (MG)

MG is a systemic autoimmune condition where there are antibodies that block receptors, preventing acetylcholine from binding and leading to a breakdown in communication between the nervous system and the muscle, resulting in muscle fatigue and sometimes paralysis. In about 25% of MG patients, the initial manifestation is nonocular. Do not offer IOL monovision to those who carry this diagnosis even if they "never had eye problems before," because about 90% of MG patients eventually have eye involvement. Besides ptosis and any form of diplopia, it can cause gaze-evoked nystagmus.

Multiple Sclerosis (MS)

MS is another systemic condition that should contraindicate IOL monovision. The most common ocular involvement is probably optic neuritis, but double vision and abnormal eye movement including nystagmus and internuclear ophthalmoplagia are not rare presentations.

History of Cranial Nerve Palsy

For patients with a history of a cranial nerve palsy and a short period of double vision, such as third, fourth, or sixth nerve palsies, we probably should not offer IOL monovision, even if they do not have any manifest residual EOM misalignment. The concerns are mainly twofold: the EOM system may

still have some subtle dysfunction and the palsy may recur because of their systemic conditions.

Meniere's Disease

Meniere's disease is likely not an absolute contraindication for IOL monovision, but it can be a reason for caution. The vestibular system includes the parts of the inner ear and brain that process sensory information controlling balance and eye movements. If disease or injury damages these processing areas, vestibular disorders can result. Meniere's disease is one of the most commonly diagnosed vestibular disorders. It is probably advisable to avoid IOL monovision for any patient who has had a repeated history of vertigo episodes because those diseases are often chronic in nature. Monovision itself may not necessarily make Meniere's disease worse, but an extra anisometropic load may make balance and visual system function more complicated and be blamed as the etiology.

4.8.4 Other Contraindications and Concerns

The profession and avocations of monovision candidates should always be considered. Some professions may require perfect stereovision and we may need to avoid IOL monovision for those patients. One medical-legal case was reported[79] of an airplane accident related to contact lens monovision in a pilot. The practitioner was not aware of the occupation of the patient. Truck drivers and professional athletes such as basketball, tennis, baseball, and golf players may not be ideal candidates for full monovision.

Significant corneal astigmatism is not a contraindication for IOL monovision, but without correcting severe cornea astigmatism, IOL monovision may not work.[41] There is no agreement as to what should be considered a "significant" amount of astigmatism for pseudophakic monovision. Our experience suggests that the maximum astigmatism for the distance eye should be less than 0.50 D to 0.75 D and for the near eye about 1.25 D to 1.50 D, the less the better. Leaving a small amount of with the rule astigmatism might be better in the long term, since, as patients age, horizontal astigmatism is likely to gradually worsen.

One common mistake in IOL monovision is when surgeons assume that all patients want to have spectacle independence. Our own clinical survey noted that about 50% of cataract patients did not want to have any presbyopia management at the time of cataract surgery, although the rate would be expected to be much lower than 50% if financial concerns were not counted. If a patient does not like the idea of one eye for far and one eye for close, or if a patient would like to have glasses for other reasons, then we should not offer IOL them monovision.

4.8.5 Summary of Pseudophakic Monovision Contraindications

Any patient with history of strabismus, EOM surgery, prism usage, double vision, tropia or significant phoria should not be considered as an IOL monovision candidate. Longstanding dense unilateral cataract eyes probably should not be considered for IOL monovision, especially crossed monovision. It is best to avoid monofixation syndrome and amblyopia for monovision, especially crossed IOL monovision. Patients with severe ocular comorbidities do not do well with IOL monovision. Some systemic conditions, such as Parkinson's disease, Graves's disease, myasthenia gravis, and multiple sclerosis are relative contraindications for IOL monovision.

4.9 Who Should Be My First Few IOL Monovision Patients and How Should I Start My First Case?

Patient motivation is the number one factor. If a patient prefers to have glasses as an integral part of their appearance to hide skin wrinkles or for whatever reasons, there is no point in offering them IOL monovision. Choose someone with a strong desire to decrease their dependence on glasses.

Just like other routine cataract patients, preoperative hyperopic patients typically have a high postoperative satisfaction rate because they could not see far or near without glasses before the surgery, while myopic patients often do not have much of a problem for near without glasses. You may wish to avoid high hyperopia for your first few patients. For very short or very long eyes, effective lens position can be a concern. For myopic patients who now need cataract surgery, it is important if you offer and they choose IOL monovision, that you warn them of the possibility of their postoperative near vision with or without glasses not being as good as their preoperative

near vision. As Dr. Fonda mentioned in his book *Management of Low Vision*[80]: "Myopia patients have a built in magnifier in their eyes which often makes them see very well at near. You may need to mention to these myopic patients that the reading distance after surgery may be different from their preoperative habitual reading distance."

If the patient has significant corneal astigmatism, make sure that it is correctable (not irregular) and that the patient is willing and able to pay the cost if indicated. It is desirable to have the dominant eye 20/20 to 20/30 uncorrected after surgery in order to have a really good IOL monovision outcome; that means the distance eye should be emmetropic or near –0.25 D. The nondominant eye has relatively more leeway in terms of astigmatism as well as myopic defocus end point. We have sometimes noted no significant impact on patient satisfaction even when the near eye has about 1.00 D to 1.50 D of residual astigmatism.

Patient satisfaction is a relatively subjective combination of many factors. A patient with an easygoing personality will make your first few IOL monovision cases much easier.

It is advisable to start with mini- or modest monovision with an anisometropic level of about 1.00 D to –1.50 D rather than 2.00 D or higher. Tell these patients that "I am going to aim at good distance vision but also cover arm's length vision, such as the dashboard, computer and casual reading for your smart phone, but you may still need glasses for reading small print." For these patients, you will hardly have any issues at all if you hit the targets. Those patients are almost always happy. As one gets more experience, you can gradually increase the anisometropic amount for those patients who desire good small print coverage. Typically, full monovision patients with anisometropia of 2.00 D will not need readers, but there is the downside of compromised near stereovision. In the real world, these patients do quite well.

One of the three most important requirements for successful IOL monovision is to avoid potential contraindications. (For details, see the section "Contraindications and Concerns.") Any patient with a history of strabismus, EOM surgery, prism usage, double vision, tropia, or significant phoria should not be considered an IOL monovision candidate. It is better to avoid monofixation syndrome and amblyopia for monovision, especially crossed IOL monovision. Patients with severe ocular comorbidities should be carefully evaluated on a case-by-case basis with attention to their suitability and scope of pathology and stability.

4.9.1 How Should I Start My First Case?

1. Find a patient who does not like glasses. A modified Dell's preoperative survey is very helpful in this regard. This survey will tell you the patient's needs, lifestyle, hobbies, and preferences. Based on this, during your consultation you can make your decision as to the amount of monovision desired.
2. Identify the dominant eye with the hole-in-card test. Make sure the card is held with both hands to avoid laterality impact.
3. Ask the patient if they have any history of double vision, prism usage, eye muscle surgery, amblyopia, etc., and do a careful cover and uncover test to avoid contraindications.
4. Set anisometropia at a modest level, about –1.0 to –1.25 D.
5. Perform a good preoperative consultation and document that you have discussed the benefits and risks of monovision. Make patients aware that there is no guarantee of complete freedom from glasses.
6. You can either do the worst cataract eye first or the nondominant eye first.
7. Conventional IOL monovision is still preferred over crossed IOL monovision.
8. The rest will be the same as what you do routinely for your cataract patients. Accurate preoperative biometry (it is highly recommended that two technicians do all the preoperative biometry, corneal photography, and manual keratometry for each patient to avoid human errors), and the ability to correct corneal astigmatism, if indicated, and hit the refractive target are very necessary.

4.9.2 Summary: Who Should My First Few Patients Be?

The following list will help you to choose your first few IOL monovision patients:
1. Those who have a strong desire for glasses independence.
2. Those who have a history of contact lens monovision, natural monovision, or laser vision correction monovision. Keeping the same monovision pattern is recommended.
3. Those who do not have significant corneal astigmatism or whom you can correct to less than –0.50 D, especially for the distance eye.
4. Preoperative hyperopic patients are easier to please.

5. Avoid very demanding personalities for your first few cases.
6. Avoid contraindications.

4.10 Premium IOLs and IOL Monovision

IOL monovision works well, but it is not perfect. It is not the summit of technology. It has been more than three decades since the first known IOL monovision study published in 1984.[1] As surgeons, we should not limit ourselves to the established successful techniques and close the door to new technology. On the flip side, we should not persist with the new techniques if they are not as good. The goal is to use the best for our patients in a professional and ethical way. Often, especially for older surgeons, it is not easy to adapt to new procedures. Historically, resistance to revolutions can be significant. Both Ridley and Kelman were severely criticized by their ophthalmology communities for many years until their innovations were improved. It took Edison hundreds of trial and error experiments before his first commercial electric light bulb. LASIK may not have become a household name if we did not previously have RK. Most new technologies take time to become optimal or near ideal situations. Surgeons have to keep open minds and be willing to try new things; but they should not stick to new things if they are not really working as well as they are claimed to, or if they are not as good as older methods. We must follow the rules of evidence-based practice. Combining IOL monovision with newer technologies can serve our patients better. One-size-fits-all does not work well.

4.10.1 Multifocal IOLs

Multifocal IOLs were designed with the purpose of improving unaided near vision and reducing overall spectacle dependence. Most patients are satisfied with the spectacle independence that these lenses provide, but they do come with some compromises: decreased contrast, dysphotopsias, high cost, and a high IOL exchange rate.

The through focus curve for monofocal lenses has a single focus for distance that provides some intermediate acuity but usually inadequate unaided near vision. A diffractive multifocal implant, in contrast, has two peaks, providing good vision for distance and near, but lacks intermediate acuity. Monovision provides an additional focus for near in the second eye and the combined through focus curve is not dissimilar to the natural accommodative lens.

A randomized study of 212 patients was done at Moorfields Eye Hospital to compare bilateral multifocal IOL versus monofocal IOL monovision.[33] That study noted a complete spectacle independence rate of 25.8% in the monovision arm and 71.3% in multifocal arm, with the anisometropic level near 1.00 D. The bilateral uncorrected distance vision did not differ significantly between the two groups, but intermediate distance vision was much better in the monovision group ($p = 0.0001$) and near vision was much better in the multifocal group ($p = 0.037$). Six patients, 10 eyes (5.7%), in the multifocal group had IOL exchange in the first year after the surgery and none in the monovision group.

Another small sample prospective cohort study[2] found very comparable results in terms of best bilateral distance vision without glasses, best bilateral near vision without glasses, and spectacle independence between the two groups. In terms of overall patient satisfaction and significant visual complaints, the monofocal IOL monovision group did better than the multifocal IOL group. The average refractive power in the near vision eye in the monovision group was –1.92 D, with a median of –1.88 D.

When multifocal IOL correction was compared with IOL monovision, the overall satisfaction rate typically was high in both groups and the bilateral unaided distance vision was typically similar.[2,3,33,39,81] When comparing unaided near vision and intermediate vision, we often see a difference. Two randomized studies comparing multifocal IOLs and IOL monovision, one by Labiris et al[39] and one by Wilkins et al,[33] have noted that multifocal IOL patients had better bilateral unaided near vision as well as statistically significantly better spectacle independence than IOL monovision patients, but the anisometropic level between the two eyes in the monovision group was less than 1.00 D in both studies.

It is interesting to speculate that one of the reasons for the dissociation between spectacle independence and patient satisfaction is that spectacles typically do not offer any improvement in reading in the absence of refractive error with a multifocal implant whereas reading glasses are helpful for almost all patients with modest monovision who may appreciate the additional assistance for particular visual tasks.

It is well documented in the literature that multifocal IOL patients have a much higher rate of dysphotopsia, difficulty with nighttime driving, glare and halo complaints when compared to IOL monovision patients.[2,33,39,48,81,82,83] Contrast is well known to be compromised in multifocal IOL patients; as has also been demonstrated by an FDA comparison study.[81] To our knowledge, there is no study showing that IOL monovision has increased dysphotopsia, glare, or halos compared to monofocal non-monovision, although a mild decrease in contrast can be a concern, especially at low illumination, such as nighttime driving.[22,56,84] (An ongoing prospective study is in process at F. Z.'s office in terms of contrast under regular daytime vs. nighttime illumination for IOL monovision patients.) For the clarity of retina fundus examination, our experience echoes a study from retinavitreous surgeons: it is more difficult to view the fundus in patients with multifocal IOLs than with monofocal IOLs.[85]

A study by Harris et al[86] with 20 ametropic/presbyopic but otherwise healthy eyes with good corrected vision and normal stereovision showed that contact lens monovision was preferred by most patients when it was compared with diffractive bifocal contact lenses. Each patient was tested when wearing each of three different soft contact lenses: (1) diffractive bifocal contact lenses, (2) monovision contact lenses, and (3) distance contact lenses combined with reading spectacles. At the end of 6-week wearing periods, the 20 participants were forced to make a choice: 18 chose to have monovision and 2 chose diffractive bifocal lenses. If we could have a similar trial comparison between multifocal IOL and IOL monovision, similar to the above-mentioned study,[86] we would probably see a similar result.

IOL monovision is more tolerant of coexisting ocular pathology than are multifocal IOLs (for details, see Chapter 5 "Ocular Comorbidities and Pseudophakic Monovision"). A mild or sometimes even moderate level of dry eye syndrome, defocus created by corneal astigmatism, IOL decentration or tilt, posterior capsule opacification, mild to moderate glaucoma without central fixation involvement, epiretinal membrane, macular degeneration, and other maculopathies will have a limited impact on IOL monovision, especially if it occurs only in the nondominant eye. In their postoperative years, patients may develop more against the rule cylinder and macular function may deteriorate with aging.

These ongoing changes will have much more impact on multifocal IOLs than on IOL monovision. Among imperfect outcomes of IOL monovision patients, i.e., uncorrected vision is 20/30 or 20/40, most seem to do very well, with high satisfaction and reasonable spectacle independence. Occupation and personality are not critical screening factors in patient selection for modest monovision. Although multifocal IOLs may well not be a good choice for discriminating individuals such as architects or engineers, these professions are acceptable candidates for modest monovision as are artists and truck drivers; if required, spectacles can be worn for activities such as night driving.

Although multifocal implants provide a high level of spectacle independence, this parameter is not the most important index for patient satisfaction and a successful outcome. We are sure that many of our colleagues have also seen patients after multifocal IOL implantation, with unaided 20/20 and J1 vision, who are highly unsatisfied, even requiring lens exchange. In contrast, IOL monovision offers a high-quality optical solution, as patients can always gain good vision with the addition of spectacles if required, which is not feasible with multifocal implants.

I (F. Z.) have shifted my refractive cataract surgery more and more toward IOL monovision as I have noted the major downsides of multifocal IOLs, especially since our comparison study[2] published in 2011. I still occasionally use multifocal IOLs, but have pretty much limited their use to those patients who do not like the concept of monovision and do not drive at night but still demand complete glasses freedom, especially at near. One of the strategies to avoid explanation is to do the nondominant eye first. If the patient is very happy, with no issues regarding dysphotopsia, then use the same multifocal for the dominant eye. If they are not happy, use a nonglistening monofocal in the dominant eye aiming for plano. This strategy works very well as long as you hit the refractive target in the dominant eye. The importance of paying close attention to *each* patient's preferred reading distance and then choosing the appropriate level of add cannot be overemphasized. Carefully check to see if there is significant irregular astigmatism or maculopathy since they are the common reasons for multifocal IOL patients' dissatisfaction.

4.10.2 Accommodating IOL

Currently the Crystalens and the Trulign Toric (Bausch and Lomb, Inc., Rochester, NY) are the only premium accommodating IOLs approved by the FDA as accommodating IOLs for cataract surgery that improve near vision by a focusing process called accommodation. The 1CU accommodative IOL of HumanOptics, Erlangen, Germany, is available in Europe and many other parts of the world, but is not FDA approved in the United States. There are three generations of Crystalens: AT50SE, HD, and AO. The Crystalens AT50SE was the first generation which had a spherical design. The Crystalens HD has a central 1.5-mm thickening which was believed to increase near vision. With the HD model, it can be a bit challenging to achieve a perfect refractive target and most surgeons now are using the third generation AO model. The Crystalens AO has an aspherical design. Astigmatism correction is integrated within the Trulign lens; otherwise the two lenses share similar characteristics in terms of appearance and functional mechanism. In an accommodating IOL, the haptics are designed to keep the IOL securely in place and prevent rotational movement, but the joints between the haptics and the optic are flexible in a way that allows the optic to move slightly forward upon contraction of the ciliary muscle.

The diameter of the Crystalens is smaller than that of most conventional monofocal IOLs, 5 mm versus 6 mm. That design alone may be helpful to increase uncorrected near vision, but the downside of a small optic is that it may not work well for patients with large pupils. This can also affect nighttime driving. One of F. Z.'s Crystalens patients needed an IOL exchange for this reason; he is doing well after IOL exchange to a conventional 6-mm monofocal IOL. We postulate that this was due to the hinged plate-haptic-to-optic junction not being well covered by the large pupil at nighttime.

The Crystalens typically requires mini-monovision to enhance the near vision. A frequently used pattern is to aim the dominant eye for plano to –0.25D and the nondominant eye for –0.50 to –0.75D as mini-monovision. Even with this approach, it is not rare for patients to need readers for small print. This is likely due to the limited accommodation level.

Though the Crystalens is designed to provide an expanded range of clear vision compared with conventional monofocal IOLs, the efficacy of expected accommodation may still be a concern. In theory, different from multifocal IOLs, an accommodating IOL should demonstrate one of the following features to achieve a refractive power change: movement of the IOL, increased curvature of the IOL, increased thickness of the IOL, or increased separation of the optics of a dual optic IOL.[87] We have seen noticeable variation in outcomes with the Crystalens. Some patients can have good uncorrected distance vision and great uncorrected near vision, but some patients hardly show any advantage in uncorrected near vision. This can be more of a concern when the implant is surrounded by ongoing stiff capsular fibrosis, which may prevent meaningful flexible accommodating movement. A recent review by Pepose et al in *Current Opinion in Ophthalmology* noted that the Crystalens and several other single optic presbyopia-correcting IOLs may be providing improved intermediate or near vision predominantly through pseudo accommodative mechanisms, in addition to small changes in axial translation.[88] Studies with a laser ray tracing aberrometer, UBM, and three dimensional OCT have demonstrated a significant frequency of paradoxical posterior optic movement during accommodative effort.[88] The Crystalens is also associated with more posterior capsule opacification and a high YAG laser capsulotomy rate.[89] A unique complication with the Crystalens is the Z-syndrome due to asymmetric capsular fibrosis and contraction causing one plate haptic to move anteriorly and one posteriorly. Mild forms of Z-syndrome can be managed with the YAG laser, but severe Z-syndrome typically requires explantation and exchange or severe astigmatism will remain.

4.10.3 Extended Depth of Focus (EDOF)

Positive corneal aberrations can compromise retinal image quality and cause glare and halos.[90] A study of 504 elderly patients has demonstrated that the total corneal spherical aberration (SA) in the cataract population (age 60–90 years old) was in the range of 0.360 to 0.476 µm.[91] The average SA of the anterior corneal surface was 0.361 ± 0.122 at age 60 to < 70, 0.401± 0.139 in the 70 to < 80 group and 0.440 ± 0.145 in the 80 to 90 group. Significant differences were observed among the 3 age groups. A study of 134 refractive surgery and cataract patients with a mean age 50 years ± 17 (SD), range 20 to 79 years, demonstrated mean total SA of the anterior cornea of 0.281 ±0.086 µm.[92] That study[92] did not reveal an age trend for SA, although it did find that the root mean square (RMS) of total higher order aberrations (HOA) and coma correlated positively with increasing age.

Different from diffractive MF IOLs, which split the incoming light to create both distance and near focal points, EDOF lenses provide a continuous range of vision from distance through intermediate and into near. In our modern lifestyle involving the use of computers, smart cell phones and tablets, EDOF provides good coverage for these functions while maintaining good contrast quality comparable to monofocal IOLs. EDOF IOLs have an achromatic diffractive pattern that elongates the focus and compensates for the chromatic aberration of the cornea.[93] The Tecnis Symfony IOL (Johnson and Johnson Vision) also has -0.27 µm spherical aberration (personal communication with Tecnis Symfony team, J&J Vision) to compensate for corneal positive aberration. The aberration correction mechanism, together with the diffractive design, provides an elongated focal length, so no distinct out-of-focus images generating halos are present. This might explain the low incidence of photic phenomena. EDOF has better contrast sensitivity, less halo/glare and better tolerability than traditional multifocal IOLs. Due to the reduction of positive spherical aberration, the Tecnis Symfony IOL may not be the best option for patients with a history of hyperopic LASIK from a spherical aberration perspective.

A study of 411 bilateral Symfony IOLs in Europe reported by Cochener et al[93] noted that the level of satisfaction was very high: More than 91% of patients would recommend the same procedure to their friends and family, and up to 94% would choose the same IOL again. For the whole group, glasses freedom was 74.5% never/occasionally needed glasses for near activities, and 14.4% frequently needed glasses for near. In terms of incidence and level of photic phenomena at 4- to 6-month follow-up, 6.6% complained of moderate and 3.1% of severe halos; 5.0% had moderate and 2.0% severe glare. None needed explantation by 4- to 6-month follow-up. That study also compared outcomes between the non-monovision and the monovision group. The monovision group, with the nondominant eye aimed at –0.50 to –0.75 D with mean –0.75 D and SD of ±0.52 D, had 112 patients. The non-monovision group, bilaterally emmetropia, had 299 patients. The monovision group had better outcomes. The improvement in UNVA (p = 0.01), UIVA (p = 0.003), and near spectacle independence was associated with a significantly higher level of satisfaction in the monovision group. This result suggested that the Tecnis Symfony IOL with EDOF design still needs minimonovision to enhance near vision. Together with a mini level of monovision, this implant can increase the level of spectacle independence while retaining the "blended" or binocular nature with less impact on stereoacuity. Many surgeons find that the combination of mini- or modest monovision with the extended depth of focus Symfony IOL greatly improves near vision.

Thus far, our limited experience (since FDA approval in fall of 2016 in the United States) with the Symfony EDOF IOL has been good in terms of patient satisfaction and glasses independence, although most patients still have some mild glare and halo during nighttime driving. It seems to be more forgiving in terms of residual astigmatism and lens centration. EDOF is not an accommodating IOL, so the amount of increased depth of focus is limited. It is still a very common practice to use some mini-monovision to achieve better glasses independence.

4.10.4 Toric IOL

Astigmatism is a common condition. An estimated 47% of the European population between the ages of 8 and 70 have 0.75 D or greater and more than a third of the population have more than 1 D.[94] A large cataract survey keratometry database shows that greater than 60% of patients had 0.75 diopters of corneal astigmatism or more prior to cataract surgery.[95] IOL monovision may not work if significant astigmatism is not effectively corrected.

When the cornea has significant regular astigmatism in a cataract patient, the two most common intraoperative modalities employed during cataract surgery are toric IOLs and LRIs. LRI has been commonly used and is easy to perform and costs less than a toric IOL, but it can provide acceptable results rather than precision. Many studies have suggested more predictable outcomes and better durability with toric IOLs than with LRI.[96,97,98,99] Among the following new technologies, toric, aspheric, edge designs, and multifocality/bifocality, toric optics was ranked most important with the best performance by more than 800 email surveys among *Review of Ophthalmology* readers in 2016.[100] Toric IOLs are the most commonly used premium IOLs in cataract surgery.

The discovery of the noticeable impact of astigmatism from the posterior cornea on total corneal astigmatism by Koch and his colleagues has improved the clinical outcomes of toric IOLs.[101,102] Newer IOL calculation formulas that take into account the effect of the posterior cornea in toric IOL calculations, such as the Barrett Toric Calculator, have also significantly improved clinical outcomes, resulting in significantly lower levels of residual refractive cylinder than might be expected with standard calculators.[103,104,105] With the advent of the Barrett Toric Calculator, the necessity of instruments such as the Pentacam to evaluate the astigmatism of the posterior cornea has become less important.[105,106] This is a significant advantage to those who may not have the capital required to keep up with all the new expensive tools for routine refractive cataract surgery. Hopefully, technology with direct measurement will become easier and get better accuracy in the near future.

We need to accurately measure the amount of corneal astigmatism, since total refractive astigmatism may include a lenticular component. We typically use several instruments in our office to evaluate corneal astigmatism, such as the manual keratometer, IOL Master or LenStar, corneal topographer, etc. We are not able to get exactly the same results when those instruments are used to evaluate the same eye because different equipment is designed to measure different locations and diameters. Studies to date have yet to determine which one has had the highest accuracy and repeatability.[107] Then how should we decide how much astigmatism to correct and what the axis should be? One rule of thumb is to lay out all of the printouts on a table, including the patient's current spectacle refraction. The average level of cylinder is usually considered. The axis of cylinder in the patient's glasses should be considered to be as important as the instrument measurements if the level of astigmatism is great enough. The axes are expected to be very close to each other if the astigmatism is regular, although the astigmatism amplitude and axis on the glasses are for total astigmatism, including the posterior cornea and lenticular astigmatism. Not all of these measurements should bear equal weight. For example, manual keratometry has its limitation of 4 points of data and it is not able to tell you irregular astigmatism digitally. It is also almost impossible to detect peripheral abnormalities, such as keratoconus. On the other side, the printout of the LenStar and the new IOLMaster 700 with the newer version of the Barrett Toric Calculator should bear more weight since the posterior cornea and the impact of the corneal incision are already taken into account. With the assistance of intraoperative aberrometry, such as the ORA, we can expect to place most of our toric IOLs in an accurate position. If the measured axes from these different instruments are far apart, and if the measurements were accurate and ocular surface conditions acceptable, that will typically tell us either there is no or very low astigmatism, or irregular astigmatism and no toric IOL should be considered.

It is very easy to miss irregular astigmatism. We know that an optimal ocular surface and healthy retina are almost imperative for almost all premium IOLs in order to have good outcomes. Irregular astigmatism and macular pathology can be easily missed if we do not routinely do corneal topography and macular OCT. Make it a routine to check for anterior basement membrane dystrophy and dry eye in every single patient, including your conventional cataract surgery, otherwise it can be missed. For example, a patient may call you back to change the decision to go ahead with a premium IOL, but you just did a conventional examination as for monofocal IOL without paying any attention to the details, as for premium IOL candidates. Unless you have this patient come back to repeat all the examinations and tests, you may risk missing key factors necessary for success. Macular pathology is relatively hard to miss if one does a careful slit lamp examination and a routine OCT, assuming that the cataract is not too dense, but corneal irregular astigmatism can be tough to detect unless you do a good topography exam. On slit lamp examination, the cornea can look normal. It is not rare to find some missed irregular corneal astigmatism in those unsatisfied patients. Great corrected near vision, or great pinhole vision, or great PAM (potential acuity meter) vision are valuable indicators of macular health, but the patient may still have irregular corneal astigmatism which will not give good uncorrected distance vision. So, great near vision should not be considered as a generalized indicator of a great outcome. It can be, but that is not guaranteed.

Residual astigmatism can occur for a variety of reasons: preoperative measurement errors, calculation mistakes, surgical induction, intraoperative misalignment and postoperative rotation, etc. If one does not have their typical surgically induced astigmatism included in the calculations, or the formula used does not account for posterior corneal astigmatism, then the postoperative outcome may have greater variation. Each 1-degree rotation away from the intended axis will reduce the effect of astigmatism correction by about 3% and may also induce higher order aberrations. A European review summarized 20 studies from 2000 to 2011 and noted that 11.37% of eyes still had more than 1.0 D and 30.25% more than 0.5 D of residual stigmatism after toric IOLs.[108] If realignment of the toric IOL is necessary, the Berdahl and Hardten calculator (http://astigmatismfix.com) can be very helpful. This back-calculator is also available at the ASCRS web site listed as the Toric Results Analyzer.

The tour given by Dr. Berdahl included on the web site is very helpful.

Unintentional postoperative rotation may be more likely to happen when the capsular bag is large, such as in high myopia. To prevent rotation in this situation as in large eyes, a Henderson intracapsual tension ring (Morcher GmbH of Stuttgart, Germany) may be helpful thanks to its uneven contour. Optic capture by the anterior capsular rim is another way to stabilize the IOL.

With a few exceptions, such as the Trulign IOL and Tecnis Symfony ZXT toric lenses, other conventional toric IOLs do not add extra spherical power in terms of accommodation and depth of focus other than pseudo-accommodation. However, if we combine toric IOLs with IOL monovision, we can typically achieve great clinical results with spectacle independence and patient satisfaction.

4.10.5 Light Adjustable Lens

On November 23, 2017, the light adjustable lens (LAL) from RxSight (Aliso Viejo, CA), formerly Calhoun Vision. Inc., was approved by the U.S. Food and Drug Admiration.[109] The RxSight IOL is made of a unique material that reacts to UV light, which is delivered by the Light Delivery Device, typically 2 to 3 weeks after the cataract surgery. Patients receive three to four light treatments over a period of 1 to 2 weeks, each lasting about 40 to 150 seconds, depending on the amount of adjustment needed. Light-adjustable lenses are different from others because they contain special materials, known as macromers. These materials are biocompatible with the human eye and sensitive to ultraviolet light of a specific wavelength. Macromers undergo changes when they are stimulated by this light. This process is known as photo polymerization. This involves a change in the shape of the lens and as a result, in its power. This light adjustable lens has been available outside of the United States for quite a few years and clinical studies have demonstrated good outcomes.

We welcome this LAL because this will likely lift the popularity of IOL monovision further. Once one postoperative eye is already great for far without glasses, if the patient wants to have the second eye on target for intermediate or near, that becomes possible postoperatively with this technology. With the adjustability, we can tell our patients with some certainty that we can make that happen. Another advantage is that we can customize the myopic defocus for each patient in terms of what is the best reading power he or she would like. The opposite is also true, if one's postoperative eye is great for near without glasses, we can adjust the second eye for far without much worry about not being able to hit the target, doing so without invasive laser vision correction. The LAL will also decrease the stress of preoperative patient consultation, for both the patient and the surgeon, in terms of uncertainty and how much anisometropic level to choose because of its flexibility and adjustability.

Numerous peer reviewed studies have shown that the light adjustable lens is a precise, effective, predictable, and safe technology.[110,111,112,113,114] Both the spherical and cylindrical correction ranges were shown to be up to 1.75 to 2.25 D[110,111,112,113] and the light adjustable IOL irradiation protocol seemed to be safe for corneal endothelial cells.[114]

The only reservation we have at this point is that the curing regime is cumbersome. We do not believe that refractive stability is always achieved at 2 weeks post-op, which is the designated time for lock in of refraction. This may limit the use of this technology. From this perspective, femtosecond laser adjustment does not have these limitations but it is only investigational at this stage.

4.10.6 Which One to Choose for Which Patient?

Combinations of IOL monovision, multifocal, toric, accommodating, and extended depth of focus (EDOF) IOLS and femtosecond laser assisted cataract surgery (FLACS) can provide the surgeon many options to serve a variety of patients. When a patient comes for cataract evaluation and expresses a desire for spectacle independence, how do you decide which modality to use for which patient? The following is a list of considerations:

1. If a patient does not want to spend too much out of pocket money or is unable to afford the cost, IOL monovision will be likely the best option. If we explain to our patients how high the rate of satisfaction is, by far most of them tend to choose this modality, particularly if the patient has family members, friends, or neighbors who are happy with IOL monovision. Overall, the majority of our refractive cataract surgery patients fall into this category.

2. If a patient has corneal regular astigmatism of 1.25 D or more, a toric IOL will be the best option.

3. If a patient does not drive much at night, but has a strong desire and priority for glasses freedom for reading, a multifocal IOL can be a reasonable option if the patient fully understands and accepts the concept of decreased contrast.

4. If a patient has concerns about compromised stereopsis for monovision, currently the Tecnis Symfony EDOF seems to be the best option. The results of EDOF have been very encouraging so far. It is very rare for patients with mini-monovision to experience stereopsis issues. But if a patient does not want to deal with any nighttime dysphotopsias, we should be very cautious with use of an EDOF IOL.

5. A reasonable approach in using the Crystalens is to consider a traditional monofocal IOL for the dominant eye because the conventional monofocal IOL seems to be more predictable and there is no chance of developing a Z-syndrome; the nondominant eye is then operated on with a Crystalens aiming for –0.50 D to –0.75 D. We cautiously predict that the Crystalens will be largely replaced by the Tecnis Symfony EDOF lens over the next few years.

6. If a patient has a demanding personality, IOL monovision likely will be a better option than the others. Using the priority approach is another helpful supplement to achieve patient happiness. (See details in the section "Which Eye to Operate upon First?")

7. If a patient needs an LRI and a premium IOL, femtosecond laser assisted cataract surgery (FLACS) is a great option given the fact that we do not have low level Toric IOL in the US. FLACS can also provide a perfect continuous curvilinear capsulorhexis (CCC). An imperfect CCC sometimes can affect clinical outcomes. If the CCC does not cover 100% of the optic edge, it can cause astigmatism, especially when the vitreous pressure is very high by the end of cataract surgery, pushing the IOL forward and resulting in a slightly tilted optic; postoperative capsular fibrosis may also cause IOL tilt if the CCC does not cover 100%; if the CCC is too small, it can cause increased surgical difficulty intraoperatively and future phimosis; if the CCC is too big, it can affect the effective lens position (ELP). Too big a CCC is also associated with a higher rate of posterior capsular opacification.[115]

8. If a patient has Fuchs corneal dystrophy or compromised zonules, FLACS also may have value, although we usually do not recommend premium IOLs in these cases.

4.10.7 How to Use Monovision Skills to Enhance Premium IOL Outcomes?

Mini-Monovision

This strategy mainly applies to accommodating and EDOF IOLs. The Crystalens and Symfony lens are the two typical samples. The most commonly used pattern is to aim the dominant eye for plano to –0.25 and the nondominant eye for –0.50 to –0.75 D.

Crossed Mini-Monovision

This is an underused strategy unless one knows the value of crossed monovision and knows what to avoid. What if you operate on the nondominant eye first, aiming at –0.75D with a Crystalens or a Tecnis Symfony lens but it does not end up at –0.75 D? Instead, it ends up at plano or –0.25 D with satisfactory uncorrected distance vision of 20/20 or 20/25, but uncorrected near vision of only J5. Would you consider using the same lens for the dominant eye aiming for plano and asking your patient to use readers for near? Or would you consider using the same lens aiming for –0.75 as crossed mini-monovision? If you do decide to use crossed mini-monovision, will this work? Should you have any concerns?

Our own crossed monovision study[4] and a study from South Korea[12] have proven that crossed IOL monovision works as well as conventional IOL monovision as long as the potential contraindications are avoided and the anisometropia is kept at a modest level. There are more potential contraindications for crossed IOL monovision than for conventional IOL monovision. For details, see the sections "Potential Contraindications and Concerns for IOL Monovision" and "Crossed IOL Monovision."

Armed with the option to use crossed IOL monovision, you double the chances of achieving acceptable spectacle independence when you use accommodating and EDOF IOLs.

Achieve the Priority Goal First

This strategy seems to be helpful. During the preoperative consultation, asking your patient what is his/her priority for vision without glasses, far or near? If distance vision is the priority, then consider doing the dominant eye first. If the refractive outcome from the first eye is satisfactory, then keep the original preoperative plan for the nondominant fellow eye. If the priority is for reading, operate on the nondominant eye first, aiming for –0.50 to –0.75 D if you plan to use a Crystalens or Tecnis Symfony lens. If the first operated eye comes out with the target refraction and the patient is happy, then keep the original plan for the fellow dominant eye. With advanced biometry and intraoperative aberrometry, such as the ORA, we usually can achieve what we planned, but in case we miss the first eye target, we still have one more chance to achieve that patient's priority goal and the patient can still be happy. For more discussion about how to use the focus-on priority strategy, see details in the section "Which Eye to Operate upon First?"

4.10.8 Hybrid IOL Monovision

We can sometimes run into a situation in which one eye had cataract surgery done a long time ago with monofocal IOLs and good UCDVA or UCNVA. Traditional pseudophakic monovision has two main concerns: the distance vision of the near vision eye cannot see far clearly without glasses and there is a compromise for fine depth perception. The impact of depth perception from IOL monovision in real daily life is almost negligible for mini-monovision or modest monovision patients, but the distance vision of the near vision eye can be an issue for some patients. What can we do if a patient also wants the second eye to have good vision for near as well as for far? If the pseudophakic eye has good UCDVA, we have found that an EDOF Symfony lens aiming –0.50 D for the second eye works well. The second eye with the Symfony lens can see well for intermediate vision and often sees well for near vision, but what is more, it typically can see pretty well for distance vision. If the pseudophakic eye has good UCNVA at a –1.50 level, a Crystalens or an EDOF Symfony lens aiming at plano also works well. That is what we have called "Hybrid IOL monovision." A few cases with low power add MFIOL also seem to work well if the pseudophakic eye has a monofocal IOL with good uncorrected distance vision.

This is our anecdotal experience only. More studies with large sample sizes will be needed to verify its validation. We have tried to avoid using MFIOL in the dominant eye while the nondominant eye has a monofocal IOL for near. Our experience suggests that the visual system works better if the dominant distance vision eye has better distance vision and good contrast sensitivity.

4.10.9 Summary: Premium IOLs and IOL Monovision

IOL monovision is a premium practice itself as well as the foundation for premium IOL use. It works well for most of our refractive cataract surgery patients, but it is not perfect. We should keep an open mind on trying new technology. We should not stick to the new procedures if they prove not to be better. We need to follow evidence-based practice. The combinations of IOL monovision, toric, multifocal, accommodating, EDOF and FLACS provide us a variety of choices to serve our patient needs. The newly FDA-approved light adjustable lens will increase the popularity of monofocal IOL monovision. Our initial experience suggests that the Tecnis Symfony EDOF lens works well when it is combined with mini-monovision.

4.11 Crossed IOL Monovision

In typical clinical practice, *conventional* monovision is used most commonly, where the dominant eye is corrected for distance vision and the nondominant eye is corrected for near vision. Crossed monovision, where the nondominant eye is corrected for distance and the dominant eye is corrected for near, has rarely been reported in the literature. Much of the information about crossed monovision is from laser induced cases. To our knowledge, only two studies have been published detailing IOL induced crossed monovision.[4,12]

Conventional pseudophakic monovision works well for the management of presbyopia, with high patient satisfaction and high spectacle independence. Typically, conventional monovision is used, however, unpredicted surgical outcomes or individual clinician practice patterns, may result in crossed monovision. Preoperative testing for eye dominance may not always be definitive or accurate. Because of the nature of biometry and eye anatomy, we often miss our planned refractive target, but patients may still wish to have spectacle independence. It is fairly common practice for cataract surgeons to operate on the denser cataract or worse vision eye first, aiming for a plano refraction, and on the second eye to correct for near, as monovision, regardless of which eye is dominant.[6,76,116,117] Some such patients therefore end up with crossed monovision. It typically works very well as long as contraindications are avoided.

Crossed monovision in LASIK has been reported to work well without significant differences between conventional and crossed monovision,[34,35,37] although there is no direct comparison study in the literature.

Braun[34] et al retrospectively studied 284 consecutive LASIK patients. 172 of these patients were followed up for at least one month postoperatively. Of the 160 conventional monovision patients, 11 (6.9%) chose to reverse their monovision by enhancing the near vision eye for distance. Among the 12 crossed monovision patients, 1 (8.3%) chose to reverse the monovision by enhancing the near vision for distance.

Jain[35] and colleagues studied 144 consecutive patients, 45 years or older, who were treated with excimer laser PRK or LASIK between 1995 and 1998. Among those 144 patients, 42 had a surgical outcome of monovision. The dominant eye was identified by the "hole test." In monovision patients, the average distance vision SE, near vision SE, and anisometropia were −0.04 ± 0.27 D, −1.95 ± 0.70 D, and 1.92 ± 0.74 D, respectively. Patient satisfaction was 88%. Twenty-four (57%) patients had conventional monovision and 18 (43%) had crossed monovision. All patients with crossed monovision were satisfied with their vision. Patient satisfaction with monovision showed no relationship to gender, age at initial surgery, preoperative trial of monovision, laterality of treatment, or type of monovision. Among the 18 crossed monovision patients, there were seven unpredicted crossed monovision cases, four patients were targeted for full correction, two for monovision, and one had monovision reversed after retreatment. The seven unpredicted crossed monovision patients were satisfied with their outcomes and did not have a significantly different satisfaction rate from the 11 preoperatively anticipated crossed monovision patients.

A randomized study done in South Korea by Kim et al[12] was the first in the literature to compare conventional and crossed pseudophakic monovision. A total of 59 patients from 2009 to 2012 were enrolled, 28 as conventional and 31 as crossed monovision. The more severe cataract eye was operated first aiming for −0.50 to emmetropia for distance without consideration of motor sighting or sensory dominance. The refractive target for the fellow eye was −1.50 to −2.50 D based on each patient's activity needs. Preoperatively, the hole-in-card test was used to decide which eye was dominant. There was no sensory dominance test performed prior to the surgery. If the first operated eye was the dominant eye, that patient was assigned to the conventional group. If the first operated eye was the nondominant eye, that patient would belong to the crossed group. The mean SE for the distance eye was -0.09 D in the conventional group and –0.11 D for the crossed group; and the mean SE for the near eye was –1.43 D for the conventional group and –1.56 D for the crossed group. There were no statistically significant differences noted between the two groups in terms of UCDVA, UCNVA, BCVA, stereopsis, spectacle independence, and patient satisfaction.

A crossed IOL monovision study of 7,311 consecutive cataract surgical cases performed from 1999 to 2013 by Zhang et al was reviewed.[4] Forty-four cases of crossed IOL monovision met the inclusion criteria; 30 of them were enrolled and 14 were excluded. Of the 14 excluded, 4 declined, 4 could not be contacted, and 6 could not be matched to appropriate controls. A matched control from the same surgeon's conventional pseudophakic monovision pool was assigned to each crossed pseudophakic patient with the following matching criteria:

1. Age within 10 years.
2. Same sex.
3. Similar general health.
4. Similar life style and hobbies (divided as three subgroups: far, such as golf, sports, TV; near, such as reading, woodworking, word puzzles; and mixed.)
5. Similar preoperative refractive status, such as hyperopia, myopia, or within 1 D of emmetropia for the dominant eye.
6. Post-op uncorrected vision the same or within one line, for both distance and near.
7. Post-op sphere power within 0.50 D for distance correction.
8. Post-op astigmatism within 0.50 D.

The matching process was carried out by a research assistant. A de-identified survey was sent to each candidate. All data were collected by the research asssitant and the statistical analysis was performed by an indepent statistician.

4.11.1 Inclusion

When patients with visually significant cataracts desired postoperative spectacle independence and had good vision potential, IOL monovision was offered. Study participants had at least 0.75 diopter or more postoperative anisometropia between the two eyes; postoperative distance vision without correction 20/50 or better and near vision 20/50 or better without correction; and postoperative cylinder correction of 0.50 D or less.

4.11.2 Exclusion

1. Significant ocular comorbidities such as severe diabetic retinopathy, severe age-related macular degeneration, glaucoma with significant field loss, hemianopia with history of stroke.
2. Multifocal or accommodating IOL.
3. History of prior noncataract ocular surgery.
4. History of amblyopia or strabismus.
5. Any tropia or phoria > 10 prism diopters with cover and uncover test.
6. Vitrectomy during cataract surgery.

Mean age for each group was 72 years. There were 20 females and 10 males in each group. Mean follow-up duration was 20.2 months for the conventional group and 10.5 months for the crossed group ($p = 0.059$). Mean postoperative anisometropia was 1.19 D (SD = 0.33) for the conventional group and 1.12 D (SD = 0.26) for the crossed group ($p = 0.400$) (▶ Fig. 4.6, ▶ Fig. 4.7, ▶ Fig. 4.8,

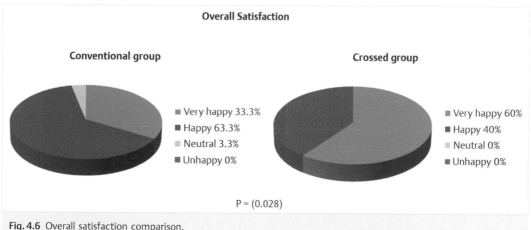

Overall Satisfaction

Conventional group

- Very happy 33.3%
- Happy 63.3%
- Neutral 3.3%
- Unhappy 0%

Crossed group

- Very happy 60%
- Happy 40%
- Neutral 0%
- Unhappy 0%

P = (0.028)

Fig. 4.6 Overall satisfaction comparison.

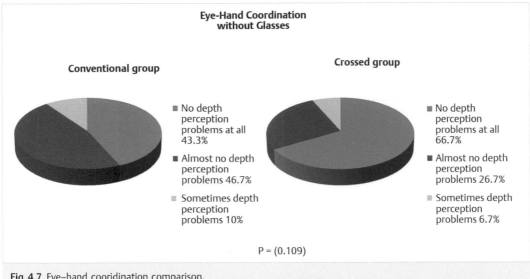

Fig. 4.7 Eye–hand cooridination comparison.

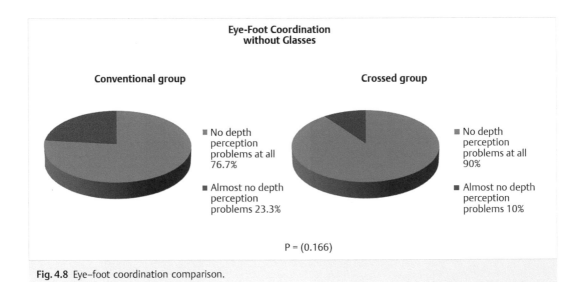

Fig. 4.8 Eye–foot coordination comparison.

► Fig. 4.9, ► Fig. 4.10, ► Fig. 4.11, ► Fig. 4.12, ► Fig. 4.13, ► Fig. 4.14, ► Fig. 4.15, ► Fig. 4.16, ► Fig. 4.17).

For overall satisfaction, glasses independence at intermediate distance and nighttime driving difficulty, the crossed monovision group did better than the conventional group with $p < 0.05$. For all other items, there were no statistically significant differences between the groups.

There is no good explanation for the fact that the crossed monovision group had better scores on some items than the conventional group in this small study. Possible explanations were: (1) small size study; (2) when deciding to elect crossed monovision, the surgeon was extra careful to make sure everything was lined up well to avoid any potential medical legal issue since that was out of "conventional" practice; (3) a few crossed monovision patients declined participating in this study for unknown reasons. Selection bias may have occurred if unhappy patients declined participation more frequently than happy ones.

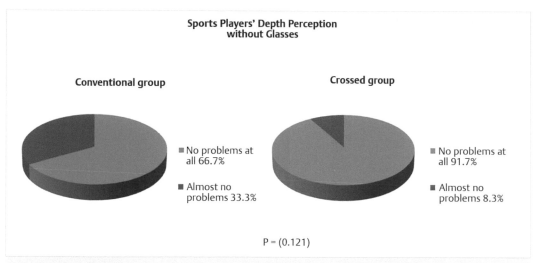

Fig. 4.9 Sports-related comparison.

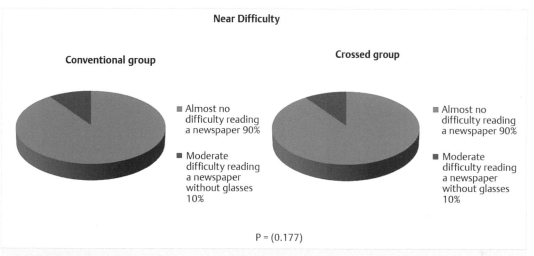

Fig. 4.10 Near difficulty comparison.

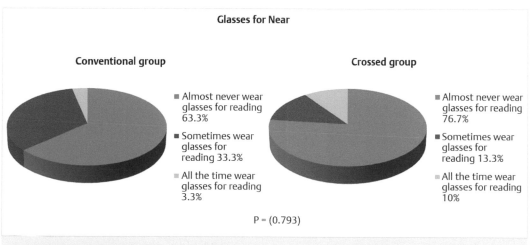

Fig. 4.11 Glasses independence for near comparison.

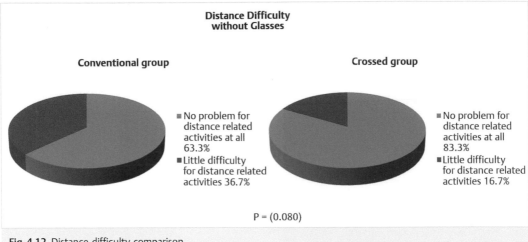

Fig. 4.12 Distance difficulty comparison.

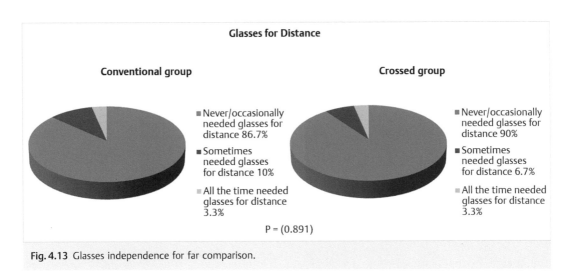

Fig. 4.13 Glasses independence for far comparison.

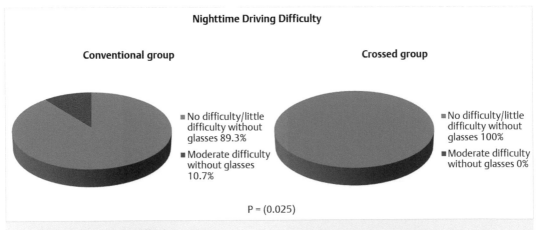

Fig. 4.14 Nighttime driving difficulty comparison.

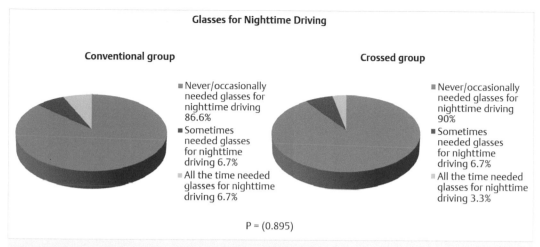

Fig. 4.15 Glasses independence for nighttime driving comparison.

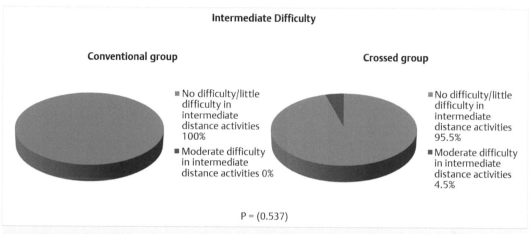

Fig. 4.16 Intermediate difficulty comparison.

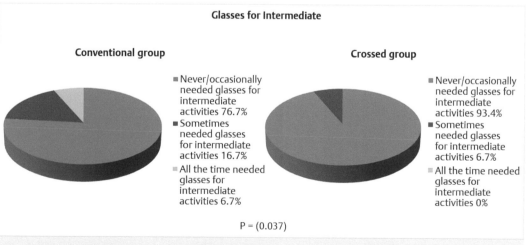

Fig. 4.17 Glasses independence for intermediate comparison.

This study demonstrated that crossed IOL monovision works as well as conventional monovision if the anisometropia level is kept at mild to modest levels and if contraindications are avoided.

Generally speaking, if possible, conventional monovision is still the preferred way to go based on the following literature data. Various advantages have been suggested in correcting the dominant eye for distance vision with the assumption that it is easier to suppress the blur in the nondominant eye than in the dominant one.[14,17,20,35,56] An experimental study with 20 healthy participants aged 20 to 28 done by Handa et al[23] noted that binocular summation was observed only after adding positive spherical lenses in the nondominant eye. The literature has suggested that correcting the sighting dominant eye for distance improved spatial locomotor activities such as walking, running, and driving,[17,20,56] and produced lesser esophoric shifts at distance.

A random and masked study of 23 presbyopic patients with normal vision and normal binocular function was studied under three conditions: both eyes fitted for distance, conventional monovision, and crossed monovision.[118] The study noted that both types of monovision (conventional and crossed) produce some stress on binocularity with small (about 1–3 prism diopters on average) esophoric shifts, but fitting the nondominant eye for distance produces more esophoric shift and greater reduction of range of vergence, although the difference was not statistically significant. The esophoric shift was also greater in the unsuccessful than in the successful patients in that study.

The nondominant eye is well suited for near tasks such as reading because these tasks do not require a precise sense of absolute visual direction.[56] Interocular blur suppression has been noted to be better in conventional monovision than in crossed monovision.[17] A contact lens fitting study with 7 successful and 12 unsuccessful monovision patients by Erickson and McGill[119] demonstrated that crossed monovision has a greater chance of affecting overall bilateral vision, reducing stereoacuity and inducing esophoria at distance when compared with conventional monovision.

Crossed monovision can cause problems in some special situations. The fusion ability can be affected at the ocular level as well as at the central nervous system level in the presence of a long history of traumatic cataracts.[69] Some ocular pathology can affect fusion ability and should be a contraindication for crossed IOL monovision. A dense cataract can present with or without an ocular deviation, as in a unilateral traumatic cataract with a long interval between the loss of vision and the restoration of vision with an IOL. While we cannot predict with certainty if those patients will do well if we correct that lesser potential eye with mild myopic defocus to increase some depth of focus, the clinical impression is that they will not do well if we happen to have that eye corrected for distance, while the healthier eye is corrected for near. My (FZ) personal preference is to correct the sighting dominant eye, which also is the healthier eye with better visual potential based on past ocular history and preoperative examination, for plano or –0.25; and the fellow "weaker" eye to be a bit more myopically defocused, at about –0.50 D if the patient wishes to have better uncorrected distance vision. If the patient prefers to have better uncorrected near vision, if their main hobbies are at near, such as reading, needlework, or word puzzles, correct the sighting dominant eye to be –1.25 to –1.50 D and the fellow "weaker" eye to the –1.50 to –1.75 D level. Correcting the eye with better vision potential by history and preoperative examination to have a bit better uncorrected distance vision seems to work best, which is consistent with what was suggested by Sheard, leaving the dominant eye with better uncorrected distance vision when spectacles are prescribed.[10,11]

The main concern with crossed IOL monovision is "fixation switch diplopia."[62,64,68,74] Crossed monovision can sometimes cause a problem if a long-suppressed eye becomes the fixating eye, especially for distance, such as an unrecognized amblyopic eye. When the longstanding suppressed eye becomes the fixating eye, whether surgically induced or spontaneously developed due to adolescent growth or due to cataract lens refractive change in adults, it may induce what is called "fixation switch diplopia." Fixation switch diplopia, discussed in the section "Potential Contraindications and Concerns for Pseudophakic Monovision," should be avoided for crossed monovision. When fixing with the preferred eye, such patients do not have diplopia, but when fixing with the nonpreferred eye, diplopia presents right away. They can show almost no symptoms when fixing with the preferred eye.

Another concern about crossed monovision is the risk of deterioration of previously balanced ocular alignment. For example, asymptomatic phorias in some monofixation and amblyopia patients can be much worse with crossed monovision than conventional monovision in terms of the extra anisometropic burden. Both can be stressful for the

EOM system and result in manifest tropias. This kind of deterioration can be the reason why some monovision patients need to wear glasses all of the time.

Detecting subtle contraindications can be a challenge for a busy surgeon, especially if the patient cannot provide a reliable ocular history, or if the cataract is very dense with very poor vision, making preoperative testing difficult or impossible. In these scenarios, it would be better not to offer IOL monovision rather than to incur the risks. Generally speaking, as long as the clinician is mindful and pays detailed attention, contraindications can be avoided. See details in the sections "Contraindications and Concerns of Pseudophakic Monovision" and "How to Detect Subtle Contraindications."

4.11.3 Summary of Crossed IOL Monovision

Crossed IOL monovision works as well as conventional IOL monovision as long as the anisometropia level is kept at a mini to modest level and potential contraindications are avoided.[4,12] Crossed IOL monovision is commonly applied in many situations such as when the first eye refractive target is missed. If possible, conventional monovision is still preferred based on extensive supporting data in the literature.

References

[1] Boerner CF, Thrasher BH. Results of monovision correction in bilateral pseudophakes. J Am Intraocul Implant Soc. 1984; 10(1):49–50

[2] Zhang F, Sugar A, Jacobsen G, Collins M. Visual function and patient satisfaction: comparison between bilateral diffractive multifocal intraocular lenses and monovision pseudophakia. J Cataract Refract Surg. 2011; 37(3):446–453

[3] Zhang F, Sugar A, Jacobsen G, Collins M. Visual function and spectacle independence after cataract surgery: bilateral diffractive multifocal intraocular lenses versus monovision pseudophakia. J Cataract Refract Surg. 2011; 37(5):853–858

[4] Zhang F, Sugar A, Arbisser L, Jacobsen G, Artico J. Crossed versus conventional pseudophakic monovision: patient satisfaction, visual function, and spectacle independence. J Cataract Refract Surg. 2015; 41(9):1845–1854

[5] Greenbaum S. Monovision pseudophakia. J Cataract Refract Surg. 2002; 28(8):1439–1443

[6] Finkelman YM, Ng JQ, Barrett GD. Patient satisfaction and visual function after pseudophakic monovision. J Cataract Refract Surg. 2009; 35(6):998–1002

[7] Ito M, Shimizu K, Amano R, Handa T. Assessment of visual performance in pseudophakic monovision. J Cataract Refract Surg. 2009; 35(4):710–714

[8] Wilkins MR, Allan B, Rubin G, Moorfields IOL Study Group. Spectacle use after routine cataract surgery. Br J Ophthalmol. 2009; 93(10):1307–1312

[9] Porac C, Coren S. The dominant eye. Psychol Bull. 1976; 83 (5):880–897

[10] Sheard C. The dominant or sighting eye. Am J Physiol Optics. 1923; 4:49–54

[11] Sheard C. Unilateral sighting and ocular dominance. Am J Physiol Optics. 1926; 7:558–567

[12] Kim J, Shin HJ, Kim HC, Shin KC. Comparison of conventional versus crossed monovision in pseudophakia. Br J Ophthalmol. 2015; 99(3):391–395

[13] Kommerell G, Schmitt C, Kromeier M, Bach M. Ocular prevalence versus ocular dominance. Vision Res. 2003; 43(12):1397–1403

[14] Seijas O, Gómez de Liaño P, Gómez de Liaño R, Roberts CJ, Piedrahita E, Diaz E. Ocular dominance diagnosis and its influence in monovision. Am J Ophthalmol. 2007; 144(2): 209–216

[15] Maloney WF. Ocular Surgery News U.S. Edition. August 1, 2005. Available at: http://www.osnsupersite.com/view.aspx?rid=18891. Accessed November 3, 2010

[16] Evans BJ. Monovision: a review. Ophthalmic Physiol Opt. 2007; 27(5):417–439

[17] Jain S, Arora I, Azar DT. Success of monovision in presbyopes: review of the literature and potential applications to refractive surgery. Surv Ophthalmol. 1996; 40(6):491–499

[18] Handa T, Mukuno K, Uozato H, et al. Ocular dominance and patient satisfaction after monovision induced by intraocular lens implantation. J Cataract Refract Surg. 2004; 30(4): 769–774

[19] Ito M, Shimizu K, Iida Y, Amano R. Five-year clinical study of patients with pseudophakic monovision. J Cataract Refract Surg. 2012; 38(8):1440–1445

[20] Schor C, Erickson P. Patterns of binocular suppression and accommodation in monovision. Am J Optom Physiol Opt. 1988; 65(11):853–861

[21] Ambati BK, Strauss L, Azar DT. Preoperative optical considerations in LASIK: refractive errors, monovision, and contrast sensitivity. In: Azar DT, Koch DD, eds. LASIK: Fundamental, Surgical Techniques, and Complications. New York, NY: Marcel Dekker; 2003:101–110

[22] Collins MJ, Goode A. Interocular blur suppression and monovision. Acta Ophthalmol (Copenh). 1994; 72(3): 376–380

[23] Handa T, Shimizu K, Mukuno K, Kawamorita T, Uozato H. Effects of ocular dominance on binocular summation after monocular reading adds. J Cataract Refract Surg. 2005; 31(8):1588–1592

[24] Charnwood L. Observations on ocular dominance. Optician. 1949; 118:85–96

[25] Khan AZ, Crawford JD. Ocular dominance reverses as a function of horizontal gaze angle. Vision Res. 2001; 41(14): 1743–1748

[26] Schwartz R, Yatziv Y. The effect of cataract surgery on ocular dominance. Clin Ophthalmol. 2015; 9:2329–2333

[27] Schor C, Carson M, Peterson G, Suzuki J, Erickson P. Effects of interocular blur suppression ability on monovision task performance. J Am Optom Assoc. 1989; 60(3):188–192

[28] Pointer JS. The absence of lateral congruency between sighting dominance and the eye with better visual acuity. Ophthalmic Physiol Opt. 2007; 27(1):106–110

[29] Handa T, Mukuno K, Uozato H, Niida T, Shoji N, Shimizu K. Effects of dominant and nondominant eyes in binocular rivalry. Optom Vis Sci. 2004; 81(5):377–383

[30] Ooi TL, He ZJ. Sensory eye dominance. Optometry. 2001; 72(3):168–178

[31] Suttle C, Alexander J, Liu M, Ng S, Poon J, Tran T. Sensory ocular dominance based on resolution acuity, contrast sensitivity and alignment sensitivity. Clin Exp Optom. 2009; 92(1):2–8

[32] Lopes-Ferreira D, Neves H, Queiros A, et al. Ocular Dominance and Visual Function Testing. Hindawi Publishing Corporation, BioMed Research International Volume 2013, Article ID 238943, 7 pages http://dx.doi.org/10.1155/2013/238943

[33] Wilkins MR, Allan BD, Rubin GS, et al. Moorfields IOL Study Group. Randomized trial of multifocal intraocular lenses versus monovision after bilateral cataract surgery. Ophthalmology. 2013; 120(12):2449–2455.e1

[34] Braun EH, Lee J, Steinert RF. Monovision in LASIK. Ophthalmology. 2008; 115(7):1196–1202

[35] Jain S, Ou R, Azar DT. Monovision outcomes in presbyopic individuals after refractive surgery. Ophthalmology. 2001; 108(8):1430–1433

[36] Goldberg DB. Laser in situ keratomileusis monovision. J Cataract Refract Surg. 2001; 27(9):1449–1455

[37] Reilly CD, Lee WB, Alvarenga L, Caspar J, Garcia-Ferrer F, Mannis MJ. Surgical monovision and monovision reversal in LASIK. Cornea. 2006; 25(2):136–138

[38] Farid M, Steinert RF. Patient selection for monovision laser refractive surgery. Curr Opin Ophthalmol. 2009; 20(4):251–254

[39] Labiris G, Giarmoukakis A, Patsiamanidi M, Papadopoulos Z, Kozobolis VP. Mini-monovision versus multifocal intraocular lens implantation. J Cataract Refract Surg. 2015; 41(1):53–57

[40] Ito M, Shimizu K, Niida T, Amano R, Ishikawa H. Binocular function in patients with pseudophakic monovision. J Cataract Refract Surg. 2014; 40(8):1349–1354

[41] Zhang FMD. Astigmatism correction and mini monovision/ReSTOR comparison. Paper presented at: 13th European Society of Cataract and Refractive Surgery, ESCRS; February 6–8, 2009; Rome Italy

[42] Collins M, Goode A, Brown B. Distance visual acuity and monovision. Optom Vis Sci. 1993; 70(9):723–728

[43] Richdale K, Mitchell GL, Zadnik K. Comparison of multifocal and monovision soft contact lens corrections in patients with low-astigmatic presbyopia. Optom Vis Sci. 2006; 83(5):266–273

[44] Hayashi K, Hayashi H, Nakao F, Hayashi F. Influence of astigmatism on multifocal and monofocal intraocular lenses. Am J Ophthalmol. 2000; 130(4):477–482

[45] Pesala V, Garg P, Bharadwaj SR. Image quality analysis of pseudophakic eyes with uncorrected astigmatism. Optom Vis Sci. 2014; 91(4):444–451

[46] Schuster AK, Pfeiffer N, Schulz A, et al. Refractive, corneal and ocular residual astigmatism: distribution in a German population and age-dependency - the Gutenberg health study. Graefes Arch Clin Exp Ophthalmol. 2017; 255(12):2493–2501

[47] Thill EZ. Theory and practice of spectacle correction of aniseikonia. In: Tasman W, Jaeger EA, eds. Duane's Ophthalmology [CD]. Philadelphia, PA: Lippincott, Williams & Wilkins; 2006

[48] Leyland M, Zinicola E. Multifocal versus monofocal intraocular lenses in cataract surgery: a systematic review. Ophthalmology. 2003; 110(9):1789–1798

[49] Pollard ZF, Greenberg MF, Bordenca M, Elliott J, Hsu V. Strabismus precipitated by monovision. Am J Ophthalmol. 2011; 152(3):479–482.e1

[50] Hayashi K, Yoshida M, Manabe S, Hayashi H. Optimal amount of anisometropia for pseudophakic monovision. J Refract Surg. 2011; 27(5):332–338

[51] Hayashi K, Ogawa S, Manabe S, Yoshimura K. Binocular visual function of modified pseudophakic monovision. Am J Ophthalmol. 2015; 159(2):232–240

[52] Pardhan S, Gilchrist J. The effect of monocular defocus on binocular contrast sensitivity. Ophthalmic Physiol Opt. 1990; 10(1):33–36

[53] Loshin DS, Loshin MS, Comer G. Binocular summation with monovision contact lens correction for presbyopia. Int Contact Lens Clin. 1982; 9(3):161–165

[54] Barrett GD. Monovision with monofocal IOLs. In: Chang DF, ed. Mastering Refractive IOLs: The Art and Science. Thorofare, NJ: Slack Incorporated; 2008:440–453

[55] Fawcett SL, Herman WK, Alfieri CD, Castleberry KA, Parks MM, Birch EE. Stereoacuity and foveal fusion in adults with long-standing surgical monovision. J AAPOS. 2001; 5(6):342–347

[56] Schor C, Landsman L, Erickson P. Ocular dominance and the interocular suppression of blur in monovision. Am J Optom Physiol Opt. 1987; 64(10):723–730

[57] Simpson T. The suppression effect of simulated anisometropia. Ophthalmic Physiol Opt. 1991; 11(4):350–358

[58] Trick GL, Dawson WW, Compton JR. The binocular VER: the effect of interocular luminance difference. Doc Ophthalmol Proc Ser. 1981; 27:295–304

[59] Duke-Elder S, Abrams D. System of Ophthalmology. Vol. 5. Anisometropia. St. Louis, MO: C.V. Mosby Co.; 1970:506 - waiting to have more page from library

[60] Naeser K, Hjortdal JØ, Harris WF. Pseudophakic monovision: optimal distribution of refractions. Acta Ophthalmol. 2014; 92(3):270–275

[61] Chen M, Chen M. A study of monofocal intraocular lens (Acrysof) in mini-monovision (MMV) and premium multifocal implantation of ResTOR. Clin Optom. 2010; 2:1–3

[62] Kushner BJ. Fixation switch diplopia. Arch Ophthalmol. 1995; 113(7):896–899

[63] Parks MM. Th monofixation syndrome. Trans Am Ophthalmol Soc. 1969; 67:609–657

[64] Boyd TAS, Karas Y, Budd GE, Wyatt HT. Fixation switch diplopia. Can J Ophthalmol. 1974; 9(3):310–315

[65] Henderson BA, Schneider J. Same-day cataract surgery should not be the standard of care for patients with bilateral visually significant cataract. Surv Ophthalmol. 2012; 57(6):580–583

[66] McDonald JE, Rotramel G. Integrating monovision into presbyopic intraocular lens surgery. In: Hovanesian JA, ed. Refractive Cataract Surgery. 2nd ed. Thorofare, NJ: Slack Incorporated; 2017:177–188

[67] Parks MM. The 1999 Gunter K. von Noorden visiting professorship lecture. Monovsion: the case for two binocular vision systems. Binocul Vis Strabismus Q. 2000; 15(1):13–16

[68] Pratt-Johnson JA, Tilison G. Why does the patient have double vision? In: Management of Strabismus and Amblyopia: A Practical Guide. New York, NY: Thieme Medical Publishers Inc.; 1994:242–246

[69] Pratt-Johnson JA, Tillson G. Intractable diplopia after vision restoration in unilateral cataract. Am J Ophthalmol. 1989; 107(1):23–26

[70] Ruben CM. Unilateral aphakia. Br Orthopt J. 1962; 19:39–60

[71] Weakley DR. The association between anisometropia, amblyopia, and binocularity in the absence of strabismus. Trans Am Ophthalmol Soc. 1999; 97:987–1021

[72] Buckley EG. Diplopia after LASIK surgery. At the Crossings: Pediatric Ophthalmology and Strabismus, pp 55–66. Proceedings of the 52nd Annual Symposium of the New

Orleans Academy of Ophthalmology. New Orleans, LA, USA, February 14–16, 2003. Edited by Robert J. Balkan, George S. Ellis Jr. and H. Sprague Eustis. © 2004 Kugler Publications, The Hague, The Netherlands

[73] Courtesy of David F Chang. MD. Altos Eye Physicians. Restor IOL Exchanges. Learning Lounge, AAO, November 14–17, 2015. Las Vegas, Nevada

[74] Richards R. The syndrome of antimetropia and switched fixation in strabismus. Am Orthopt J. 1991; 41:96–101

[75] Pratt-Johnson JA, Wee HS, Ellis S. Suppression associated with esotropia. Can J Ophthalmol. 1967; 2(4):284–291

[76] Courtesy of Arbisser LB. MD. Eye Surgeons Associations PC, Bettendorf, Iowa. Personal communication. July 5, 2015

[77] American Academy of Ophthalmology. 4 base-out prism test. Available at: www.aao.org/bcscsnippetdetail.aspx?id=7f6afb17-bf02–4b7f-b261-d419f9ad6a20

[78] Almer Z, Klein KS, Marsh L, Gerstenhaber M, Repka MX. Ocular motor and sensory function in Parkinson's disease. Ophthalmology. 2012; 119(1):178–182

[79] Nakagawara VB, Véronneau SJ. Monovision contact lens use in the aviation environment: a report of a contact lens-related aircraft accident. Optometry. 2000; 71(6):390–395

[80] Fonda GE. Management of Low Vision. New York, NY: Thieme-Stratton. Inc.; 1981

[81] Packer M, Chu YR, Waltz KL, et al. Evaluation of the aspheric tecnis multifocal intraocular lens: one-year results from the first cohort of the food and drug administration clinical trial. Am J Ophthalmol. 2010; 149(4):577–584.e1

[82] Harman FE, Maling S, Kampougeris G, et al. Comparing the 1CU accommodative, multifocal, and monofocal intraocular lenses: a randomized trial. Ophthalmology. 2008; 115(6):993–1001.e2

[83] McDonald JE, Deitz D. Monovision with aspheric IOLs. In: Chang DF, ed. Mastering Refractive IOLs: The Art and Science. Thorofare, NJ: Slack Incorporated; 2008:291–294

[84] Johannsdottir KR, Stelmach LB. Monovision: a review of the scientific literature. Optom Vis Sci. 2001; 78(9):646–651

[85] Bhavsar AR. Do multifocal optics compromise retinal treatment? In: Chang DF, ed. Mastering Refractive IOLs: The Art and Science. Thorofare, NJ: Slack Incorporated; 2008:866–869

[86] Harris MG, Sheedy JE, Gan CM. Vision and task performance with monovision and diffractive bifocal contact lenses. Optom Vis Sci. 1992; 69(8):609–614

[87] Glasser A, Hilmantel G, Calogero D, et al. Special Report: American Academy of Ophthalmology Task Force Recommendations for Test Methods to Assess Accommodation Produced by Intraocular Lenses. Ophthalmology. 2017; 124(1):134–139

[88] Pepose JS, Burke J, Qazi MA. Benefits and barriers of accommodating intraocular lenses. Curr Opin Ophthalmol. 2017; 28(1):3–8

[89] Ong HS, Evans JR, Allan BD. Accommodative intraocular lens versus standard monofocal intraocular lens implantation in cataract surgery. Cochrane Database Syst Rev. 2014(5):CD009667

[90] Holladay JT, Piers PA, Koranyi G, van der Mooren M, Norrby NE. A new intraocular lens design to reduce spherical aberration of pseudophakic eyes. J Refract Surg. 2002; 18(6):683–691

[91] Yuan L, Bao Y. Analysis of the corneal spherical aberration in people with senile cataract [in Chinese]. Zhonghua Yan Ke Za Zhi. 2014; 50(2):100–104

[92] Wang L, Dai E, Koch DD, Nathoo A. Optical aberrations of the human anterior cornea. J Cataract Refract Surg. 2003; 29(8):1514–1521

[93] Cochener B, Concerto Study Group. Clinical outcomes of a new extended range of vision intraocular lens: International Multicenter Concerto Study. J Cataract Refract Surg. 2016; 42(9):1268–1275

[94] Ferrer-Blasco T, Montés-Micó R, Peixoto-de-Matos SC, González-Méijome JM, Cerviño A. Prevalence of corneal astigmatism before cataract surgery. J Cataract Refract Surg. 2009; 35(1):70–75

[95] Abulafia A, Hill WE. The toric intraocular lens. In: Hovanesian JA, ed. Refractive Cataract Surgery: Best Practices and Advanced Technology. 2nd ed. Thorofare, NJ: Slack Incorporated; 2017:157

[96] Lam DK, Chow VW, Ye C, Ng PK, Wang Z, Jhanji V. Comparative evaluation of aspheric toric intraocular lens implantation and limbal relaxing incisions in eyes with cataracts and 3 dioptres of astigmatism. Br J Ophthalmol. 2016; 100(2):258–262

[97] Ouchi M. High-cylinder toric intraocular lens implantation versus combined surgery of low-cylinder intraocular lens implantation and limbal relaxing incision for high-astigmatism eyes. Clin Ophthalmol. 2014; 8:661–667

[98] Freitas GO, Boteon JE, Carvalho MJ, Pinto RM. Treatment of astigmatism during phacoemulsification. Arq Bras Oftalmol. 2014; 77(1):40–46

[99] Leon P, Pastore MR, Zanei A, et al. Correction of low corneal astigmatism in cataract surgery. Int J Ophthalmol. 2015; 8(4):719–724

[100] Bethke W. Surgeons tune in to the Symfony. Rev Ophthalmol. 2017(January):46–50

[101] Koch D. Steiner Refractive Lecture. 2017. ASCRS ASOA Symposium & Congress 2017. EyeWorld ASCRS NEWs. June 2017. Page 3

[102] Reitblat O, Levy A, Kleinmann G, Abulafia A, Assia EI. Effect of posterior corneal astigmatism on power calculation and alignment of toric intraocular lenses: comparison of methodologies. J Cataract Refract Surg. 2016; 42(2):217–225

[103] Gundersen KG, Potvin R. Clinical outcomes with toric intraocular lenses planned using an optical low coherence reflectometry ocular biometer with a new toric calculator. Clin Ophthalmol. 2016; 10:2141–2147–. eCollection 2016

[104] Abulafia A, Koch DD, Wang L, et al. New regression formula for toric intraocular lens calculations. J Cataract Refract Surg. 2016; 42(5):663–671

[105] Abulafia A, Hill WE, Franchina M, Barrett GD. Comparison of methods to predict residual astigmatism after intraocular lens implantation. J Refract Surg. 2015; 31(10):699–707

[106] Koch DD. The enigmatic cornea and intraocular lens calculations: The LXXIII Edward Jackson Memorial Lecture. Am J Ophthalmol. 2016; 171:xv–xxx

[107] Lee H, Kim TI, Kim EK. Corneal astigmatism analysis for toric intraocular lens implantation: precise measurements for perfect correction. Curr Opin Ophthalmol. 2015; 26(1):34–38

[108] Visser N, Bauer NJ, Nuijts RM. Toric intraocular lenses: historical overview, patient selection, IOL calculation, surgical techniques, clinical outcomes, and complications. J Cataract Refract Surg. 2013; 39(4):624–637

[109] FDA. FDA approves first implanted lens that can be adjusted after cataract surgery to improve vision without eyeglasses in some patients. Available at: https://www.fda.gov/NewsEvents/Newsroom/PressAnnouncements/ucm586405.htm

[110] Hengerer FH, Hütz WW, Dick HB, Conrad-Hengerer I. Combined correction of axial hyperopia and astigmatism using the light adjustable intraocular lens. Ophthalmology. 2011; 118(7):1236–1241

[111] Hengerer FH, Dick HB, Conrad-Hengerer I. Clinical evaluation of an ultraviolet light adjustable intraocular lens

implanted after cataract removal: eighteen months follow-up. Ophthalmology. 2011; 118(12):2382–2388

[112] Hengerer FH, Conrad-Hengerer I, Buchner SE, Dick HB. Evaluation of the Calhoun Vision UV Light Adjustable Lens implanted following cataract removal. J Refract Surg. 2010; 26(10):716–721

[113] Lichtinger A, Sandstedt CA, Schwartz DM, Chayet AS. Correction of astigmatism after cataract surgery using the light adjustable lens: a 1-year follow-up pilot study. J Refract Surg. 2011; 27(9):639–642

[114] Lichtinger A, Sandstedt CA, Padilla K, Schwartz DM, Chayet AS. Corneal endothelial safety after ultraviolet light treatment of the light-adjustable intraocular lens. J Cataract Refract Surg. 2011; 37(2):324–327

[115] Kovács I, Kránitz K, Sándor GL, et al. The effect of femtosecond laser capsulotomy on the development of posterior capsule opacification. J Refract Surg. 2014; 30(3):154–158

[116] Barrett GD. Modest monovision. ESCRS Eurotimes. 2012; 17 (5):22

[117] Barrett GD. Is monovision still an option for presbyopia? Cataract & Refractive Surgery Today. 2013:75–76

[118] McGill EC, Erickson P. Sighting dominance and monovision distance binocular fusional ranges. J Am Optom Assoc. 1991; 62(10):738–742

[119] Erickson P, McGill EC. Role of visual acuity, stereoacuity, and ocular dominance in monovision patient success. Optom Vis Sci. 1992; 69(10):761–764

5 Ocular Comorbidities and Pseudophakic Monovision

Abstract

Among elderly cataract patients, ocular comorbidity is a very common concomitant to the presence of cataracts. For those who have a very strong desire to decrease spectacle dependence, we may still consider IOL monovision as long as we provide a thorough preoperative consultation and there are no EOM related contraindications. Most mild to moderate ocular comorbidities seem to do well with IOL monovision. Some ocular pathologies may remain stable, but many can get worse post-operatively. The worsening ocular comorbidity process can be an issue for any IOL choice, but monofocal IOLs seem to have better tolerance than multifocal IOLs and EDOF IOLs. Typically, IOL monovision imposes no extra downside to the pre-existing ocular diseases from a visual function perspective as long as the patient does not have EOM and alignment disorders. Our experience suggests that most of our patients with this scenario are as happy as those who do not have ocular comorbidities. The likelihood of needing glasses in the future should be part of the preoperative consultation for all IOL monovision patients. Most patients with a history of corneal refractive surgery do well with pseudophakic monovision. Intraoperative aberrometry (such as ORA) works well in patients with a history of LASIK/PRK, but its validation in RK patients still requires more study.

Keywords: ocular comorbidity and monovision, macular degeneration and monovision, epiretinal membrane and monovision, retinal detachment and monovision, LASIK/PRK and pseudophakic monovision, RK and pseudophakic monovision, intraoperative aberrometer and IOL monovision, ORA and IOL monovision, RK and IOL monovision

5.1 Introduction

IOL monovision is predominantly used in elderly patients and age related ocular pathologies are commonly present in this population. Recent data based on more than half a million registered surgical cases from EUREQUO,[1] reported that in about 30% of patients having cataract surgery, a coexisting ocular comorbidity was present. Preexisting pathologies can get worse and new pathologies can arise as the patient ages, mainly affecting function of the macula. Unlike multifocal IOLs where optical quality and contrast loss can become more challenging when macular degeneration, epiretinal membrane, diabetic retinopathy and glaucoma field loss progress to a more severe level, IOL monovision seems to be well tolerated in most mild or even moderate situations. The single most important goal of IOL monovision is to decrease spectacle dependence. How do we match these two situations? First, they should be addressed prior to surgery. It is important to bear in mind that for those with ocular comorbidities and with a strong desire to have glasses independence, they need to understand that as they are aging, these pathologies may get worse and that they may have a greater need to wear glasses in the future. They are not ideal IOL monovision candidates to start with, but IOL monovision is likely a better option to choose than other modalities currently available. Most of these situations are contraindications for multifocal IOLs. Here are some clinical examples. (All the patients listed here have given their permission to F. Z. to use their data as was documented in their medical records.)

5.2 Case 1 Report: Status Post Retinal Detachment and Myopic Maculopathy OU

A 63-year-old woman, a practicing psychiatrist, with a history of high myopia and retinal detachment OU at age 23 had a strong desire for spectacle independence. She had a history of wearing monovision contact lenses (15 years prior to presentation) as well as multifocal contact lenses for several years until a few years ago when she developed cataracts. She did not recall any issues with either type of contact lenses. Preoperative refraction was OD –9.50 + 0.75 × 153 with distance vision 20/40 and OS –8.75 + 1.00 × 005 with vision 20/40. 2–3 + nuclear sclerotic cataracts were present in each eye with 2 + PSC OS. OD was the dominant eye. A mild macular epiretinal membrane was present OD with mild pigment changes of myopic maculopathy OU. Considering the macular changes and significant cornea astigmatism, IOL monovision was recommended rather than multifocal IOLs (▶ Fig. 5.1 and ▶ Fig. 5.2). Because of her history of happiness with contact lens monovision as well as multifocal contact lenses, a contact lens trial was ordered. (One of only two contact lens

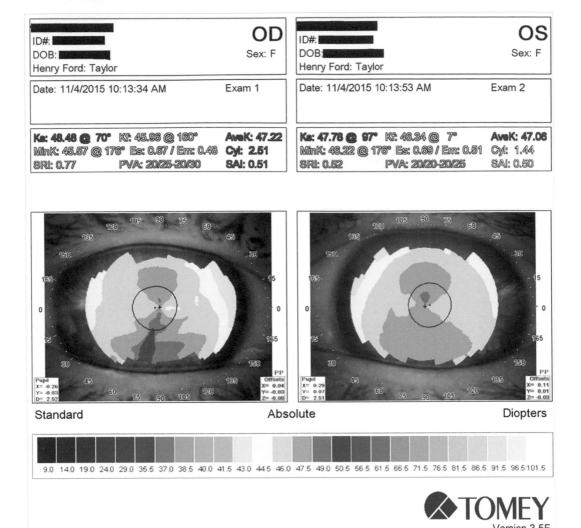

Fig. 5.1 Case 1 report. Corneal photography showing significant with the rule astigmatism. S/P retinal detachment OU and ERM OD.

trial cases in F. Z.'s two decades career using IOL monovision.) Given that her OD was always her dominant eye and was the far vision eye when she was using contact lens monovision, the decision was to aim OD for plano and OS for near, even though her OD had a mild epiretinal membrane (ERM) on OCT. Keeping the same pattern is the point. Surgery was performed with toric IOLs in OU, the left eye was treated first, followed one month later by the right. Postoperative data at 2 months: UCDVA 20/20 OD and 20/40 OS; UCNVA 20/40 OD and 20/20 OS. Refractive status: Plano OD with vision 20/20 and -1.50 sphere with vision

20/20 OS. No glasses were needed after the surgery and she was very happy (▶ Fig. 5.1 and ▶ Fig. 5.2).

5.3 Case 2 Report: S/P RK OS, ERM OU, and OAG with Field Loss OD

A 66-year-old man had a history of cataract surgery OD and 8 cut radial keratotomy OS about 20 years before his presentation. His main complaint was near vision difficulty with his OS. He strongly

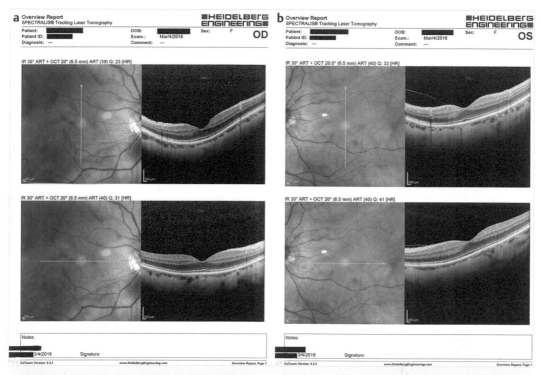

Fig. 5.2 (a,b) Case 1 report. OCT showing ERM OD. OS is unremarkable. S/P retinal detachment OU and ERM OD.

desired freedom from glasses. There were mild ERMs OU and open angle glaucoma OD with moderate field loss OD (▸ Fig. 5.3 and ▸ Fig. 5.4). Cup-to-disc ratios were 0.8 OD and 0.4 OS. The dominant eye was OD with the hole-in-card test. No other IOL monovision concerns were noted from his history and preoperative tests. Cataract surgery on OS aimed for –1.00 D. At his last office visit over 1 year later: UCDVA 20/20 OD and 20/50 OS. UCNVA J5 OD and J1 OS. Refraction: Plano OD with vision 20/20, –1.25 sphere OS with vision 20/20. He has been very happy without any glasses. More ERM was present OS, although OD had field loss with mild central fixation involvement. OS was kept for near since his OS had been used for near ever since his remote monocular RK surgery.

5.4 Case 3 Report: Epiretinal Membrane OU and Macular Pucker OD

A 72-year-old woman presented with a moderate epiretinal membrane and macular pucker OD and a mild epiretinal membrane OS (▸ Fig. 5.5).

Preoperatively the dominant eye was OS. Cataract surgery was performed on OS and 1 month later on OD. At her last visit, 4 years later, she had UCDVA 20/100 OD and 20/25 OS. UCNVA J3 OD and J3 OS. Refraction then was –2.00 + 0.50 × 025 with VA 20/20 OD and –0.50 sphere with vision 20/20 OS. She has been glasses free since the surgery.

5.5 Case 4 Report: S/P Macular Hole Repair OD and Mild Epiretinal Membrane OS

A 75-year-old woman had macular hole repair OD in 2013 (▸ Fig. 5.6, ▸ Fig. 5.7, ▸ Fig. 5.8). Preoperatively, the dominant eye with the hole-in-card test was OS. Cataract surgery was performed OD in 2014 and 2 months later OS. At her last office visit in 2016, UCDVA was 20/200 OD and 20/30 OS. UCNVA was 20/30 OD and 20/70 OS. Refraction was –1.75 sphere OD with vision 20/25 and OS –0.25 + 0.25 × 104 with vision 20/25. She stated that "I only recently started to use over the counter readers for very small print, otherwise I do not have to use any glasses."

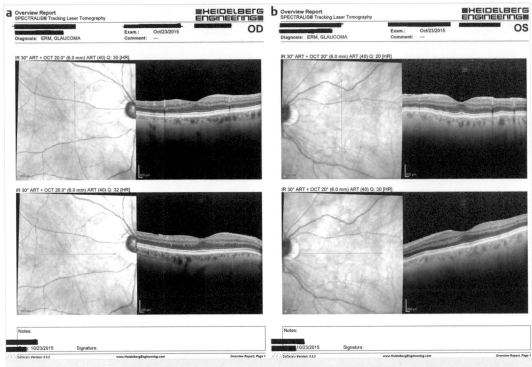

Fig. 5.3 (a,b) Case 2 report. OCT showing ERM more in OS than in OD. S/P RK OS, ERM OU and moderate field loss OD.

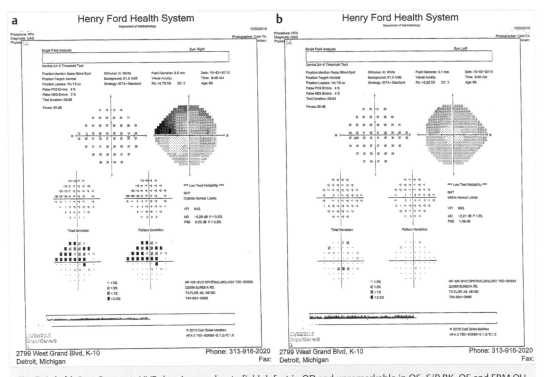

Fig. 5.4 (a,b) Case 2 report. HVF showing moderate field defect in OD and unremarkable in OS. S/P RK. OS and ERM OU, OAG with moderate field loss in OD.

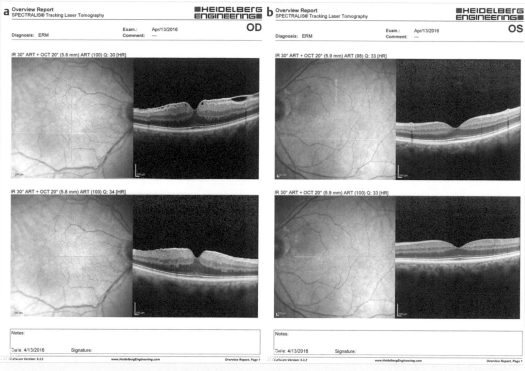

Fig. 5.5 (a,b) Case 3 report. OCT showing ERM OU and macular pucker OD.

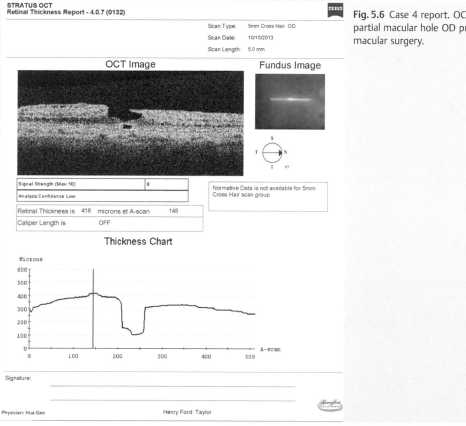

Fig. 5.6 Case 4 report. OCT showing partial macular hole OD prior to macular surgery.

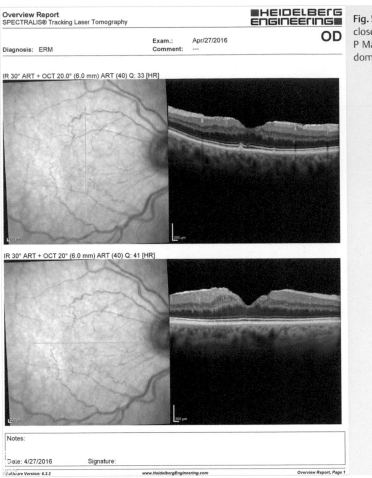

Overview Report SPECTRALIS® Tracking Laser Tomography	■HEIDELBErG ENGINEERING■

Exam.: Apr/27/2016
Comment: ---

OD

Diagnosis: ERM

IR 30° ART + OCT 20.0° (6.0 mm) ART (40) Q: 33 [HR]

IR 30° ART + OCT 20° (6.0 mm) ART (40) Q: 41 [HR]

Notes:

Date: 4/27/2016   Signature:

Software Version: 6.3.2   www.HeidelbergEngineering.com   Overview Report, Page 1

Fig. 5.7 Case 4 report. OCT showing closed macular hole with mild ERM. S/P Macular hole repair OD as non-dominant eye.

5.6 Case 5 Report: Severe AMD OU

A 75-year-old woman had severe AMD, with 3 + soft drusen OU (▶ Fig. 5.9) prior to cataract surgery. She was post LASIK OU in 1999 for myopia. She had a strong desire to be glasses free. Preoperatively OD was the dominant eye. Cataract surgery was done in 2015. At her last office visit, 8 months later, UCDVA was 20/25 OD and 20/100 OS; UCNVA was 20/100 OD and 20/20 OS. Refraction then was –0.25 sphere OD with vision 20/20 and –1.25 sphere OS with vision 20/20. She had no need for any glasses since surgery and was very happy.

5.7 Case 6 Report: Moderate Low Tension Glaucoma OU

A 69-year-old woman had low tension glaucoma in both eyes (▶ Fig. 5.10, ▶ Fig. 5.11, ▶ Fig. 5.12). Her

cup/disc ratio was 0.70 OD and 0.9 OS. She had a history of disc hemorrhage OD. A Humphrey visual field test OD was normal but OS had an inferonasal step. OD was the dominant eye prior to the surgery. She had a strong desire not to wear glasses. Cataract surgery was performed in 2012 on the left and 2 months later on the right. Her last office visit was in 2015 with UCDVA 20/20 OD and 20/70 OS; UCNVA was J16 OD and J2 OS. Refraction was plano + 0.50 × 103 with vision 20/20 OD and –1.25 sphere with vision 20/20 OS. She wore glasses as backup only for nighttime driving and very small print.

5.8 Case 7 Report: New Retinal Detachment 1 Year after IOL Monovision

A 63-year-old woman had cataract surgery OD in early 2015 and OS 2 months later for IOL

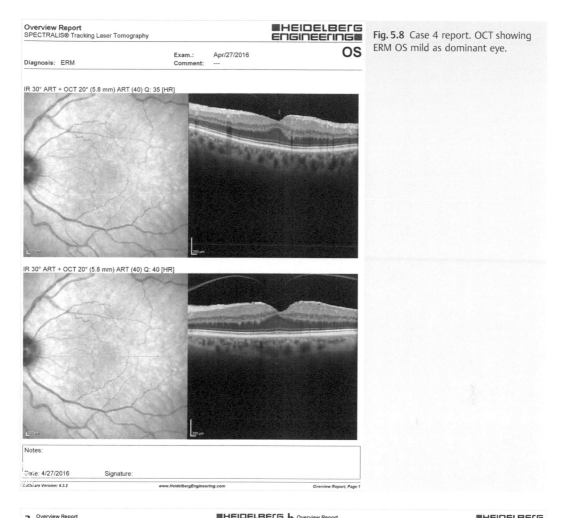

Fig. 5.8 Case 4 report. OCT showing ERM OS mild as dominant eye.

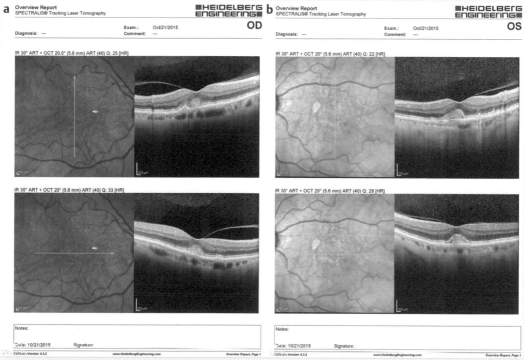

Fig. 5.9 (a,b) Case 5 report. OCT showing severe dry AMD OU.

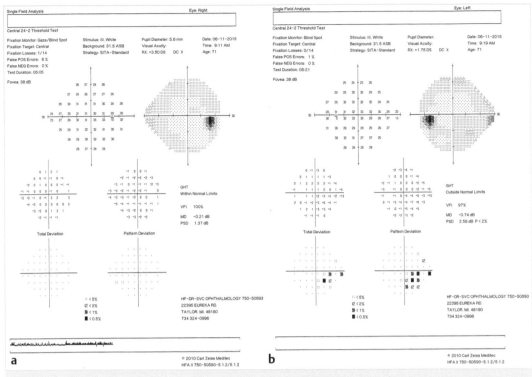

Fig. 5.10 (a,b) Case 6 report. HVF showing unremarkable OD and infranasal step OS. History of low tension glaucoma, cup/disc ratio 0.7 OD and 0.9 OS with HVF loss in OS.

monovision; OD for near and OS for far. She also had a diagnosis of glaucoma suspect with a cup/disc ratio of 0.75 OD and 0.70 OS, her highest intraocular pressure (IOP) being 23 OD and 24 OS. She was doing well until 1 year later when she had a retinal detachment of her right eye. On that day, her UCDVA was OD 20/100 and OS 20/25 +, UCNVA OD 20/30 and OS 20/100. Manifest refraction was OD −1.50 D sphere 20/20 with a supratemporal retinal detachment but her macula was still attached. Pars plana vitrectomy and endolaser were performed. At her last office visit, 6 months later, her UCDVA was 20/80 OD and 20/20 OS, UCNVA was 20/40 OD and 20/200 OS. Manifest refraction was −1.75 sphere 20/25 OD and −0.25 sphere 20/20 OS. She did have an epiretinal membrane in her right eye after retinal detachment and endo-laser treatment. IOP has been fine since cataract surgery without medications. Her field test remains full in each eye. She still does not need

any spectacles even after the onset of retinal detachment in OD.

5.9 Case 8 Report: IOL Monovision Does Not Always Work

A 78-year-old woman came for bilateral cataract surgery in 2011. On preoperative examination distance vision corrected OD to 20/50 with −1.25 + 0.50 × 040 and OS to 20/60 with −1.25 + 1.00 × 144. 3 + NS with cataract OU. She had macular drusen, very mild in OD and moderate in OS and a mild ERM in OS (▶ Fig. 5.13). Cover and uncover test showed orthophoria. OD was dominant with the hole-in-card test. The patient desired to be glasses free after surgery. Our plan was to create monovision, OD −0.25 and OS −1.50. Surgery was done on both eyes, OS first, 3 months apart. Two years later,

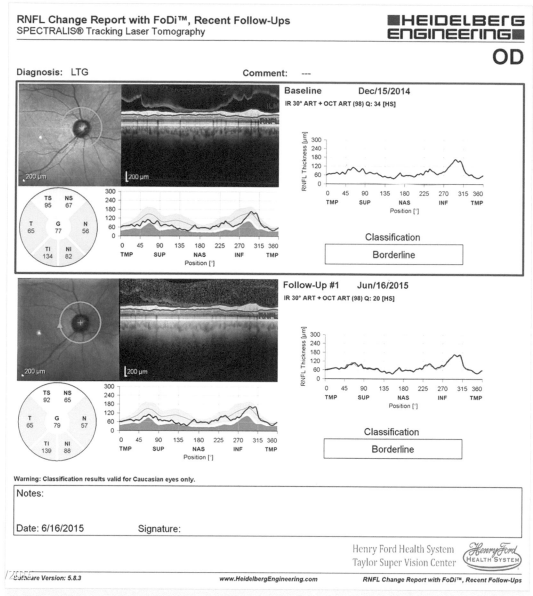

Fig. 5.11 Case 6 report. OCT OD showing superior thinning with 0.7 cup matching disc hemorrhage.

OD uncorrected distance vision was 20/40 and corrected to 20/30 with –0.25 sphere; OS uncorrected distance vision was 20/70 and corrected to 20/30 with –1.75 + 0.25 × 002. Near vision without correction was 20/40 in each eye; with + 2.50 OD 20/25 and OS 20/30. Macular degeneration was more severe than what was noted originally, although still dry in both eyes (▶ Fig. 5.14). The patient stated that she did not have to wear glasses for far, but for near, she has become more and more dependent on glasses in the last few years. She has "Never been completely glasses free."

5.10 Monovision Pearls for Previous Refractive Surgery Patients

Millions of nearsighted patients chose to get out of their glasses by having radial keratotomy (RK) in

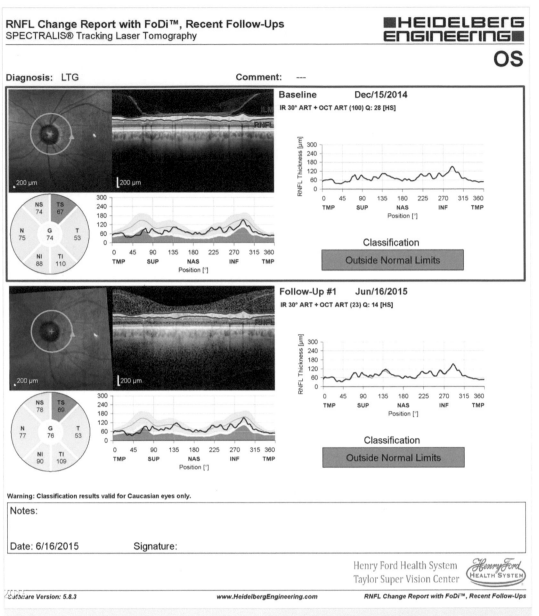

Fig. 5.12 Case 6 report. OCT showing supratemporal thinning matching HVF infranasal defect.

the 1990s. Because of delayed hyperopic regression, secondary to the loss of structural integrity of the cornea from the incisions, RK was gradually phased out and replaced by more predictable and safer laser vision correction—LASIK (laser-assisted in situ keratomileusis) and PRK (Photorefractive keratectomy). When these patients later present with cataracts they often still want to minimize spectacle dependence after cataract surgery. They

still do not like glasses or contact lenses and we often face more difficulties when they are in our offices and operating rooms. Those patients typically are motivated to have spectacle independence, but this goal can be very challenging. The challenges are focused mainly on the cornea, but we should also make sure that other parts of the eye also have the potential to meet spectacle independence as these eyes may not be as healthy as

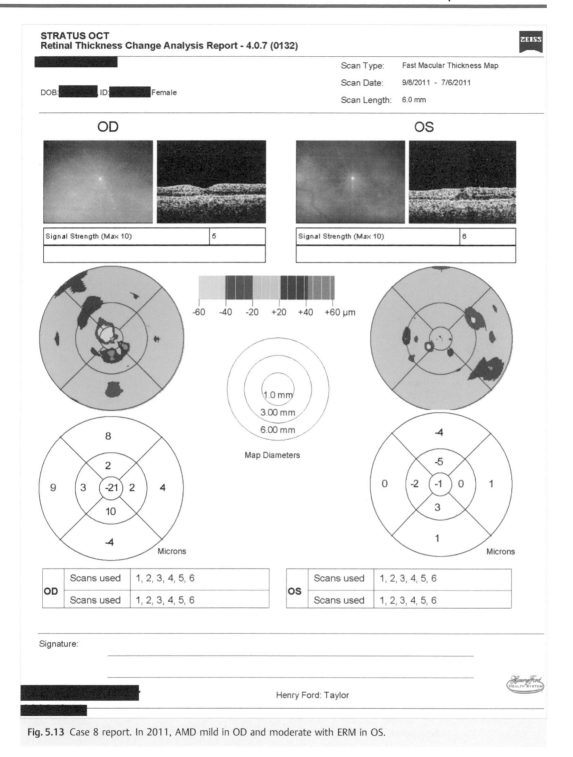

STRATUS OCT
Retinal Thickness Change Analysis Report - 4.0.7 (0132)

Scan Type:	Fast Macular Thickness Map
Scan Date:	9/8/2011 - 7/6/2011
Scan Length:	6.0 mm

DOB: ID: Female

OD

Signal Strength (Max 10) — 5

OS

Signal Strength (Max 10) — 6

-60 -40 -20 +20 +40 +60 µm

1.0 mm
3.00 mm
6.00 mm

Map Diameters

OD (Microns):
8
2
9 3 -21 2 4
10
-4

OS (Microns):
-4
-5
0 -2 -1 0 1
3
1

OD	Scans used	1, 2, 3, 4, 5, 6
	Scans used	1, 2, 3, 4, 5, 6

OS	Scans used	1, 2, 3, 4, 5, 6
	Scans used	1, 2, 3, 4, 5, 6

Signature:

Henry Ford: Taylor

Fig. 5.13 Case 8 report. In 2011, AMD mild in OD and moderate with ERM in OS.

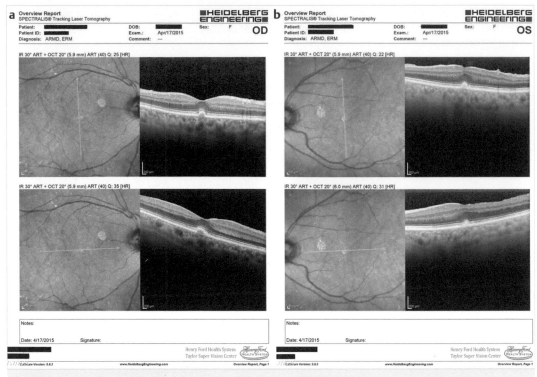

Fig. 5.14 (a,b) Case 8 report. In 2015, AMD OU and ERM OS worse than in 2011.

when they initially had corneal refractive surgery. Frequently, they are not good candidates for premium IOLs, but with IOL monovision, we can usually make them happy. The following is a list of pearls and pitfalls.

5.10.1 Preoperative Consultation

Patients should have realistic expectations. They need to know the impact of previous surgery, the complexity of the necessary IOL calculation, added intraoperative challenges due to cornea incisions, and the trend toward postoperative regression. They need to know that the outcome may not be as great as the initial "WOW vision" they experienced after their corneal refractive surgery. This is especially relevant in patients with very long or short eyes, which are not infrequent in this special group. Patients may not understand the rationale for why they have more chance of needing glasses with IOL monovision than those whose axial lengths are not extreme, but the surgeon should have a clear understanding that the effective lens position in those very short or long eyes is harder to predict even with the best IOL formulas.

5.10.2 Not All Postrefractive Surgery Patients Are Good Candidates for IOL Monovision

Those who consult based on your refractive cataract surgery reputation may not be ideal candidates for a premium IOL or monovision. Ask each RK patient whether they are aware of diurnal vision changes. Pay special attention to their corneal shape, scars, evidence of post-LASIK-ectasia, the number of RK incisions and the size and integrity of the central incision-free zone. Very irregular topography is frequently a red flag. Some severe cornea pathologies may even need referral to a cornea specialist. Severe ocular comorbidity as well as systemic contraindications also deserve your full attention.

5.10.3 Keep Their Original Monovision Pattern

Some patients were targeted for intentional monovision created by their previous RK, or LASIK/PRK procedures. Some of them were operated on in one eye only. Specifically ask them if there were any problems with their previous monovision. If they did well without any issues for a long time, try to keep the same monovision pattern regardless of the current sighting eye test for dominance. Of note, the dominant eye can change as the cataract alters vision and as post RK corneal regression progresses. A nondominant left eye can actually be the fixating eye for distance with the hole-in-card test and it is advisable to keep the OD for far and the OS for near in these circumstances. Unilateral RK was typically performed to achieve unaided distance vision, but occasionally the target could have been for near vision.

5.10.4 The Role of the Intraoperative Aberrometer

Being able to hit the refractive target is critical for the success of IOL monovision. IOL calculations in patients with a history of refractive surgery have always been a challenge for cataract surgeons. Keratometry and commonly used measurement instruments are based on an assumption that the human cornea has a fixed anterior-to-posterior curvature relationship. In patients with prior LASIK and PRK, these corneal curvature relationships have been altered. For example, in myopic LASIK corneas, the central cornea is flatter than pre-LASIK and regular measurement will overestimate the power of the cornea, resulting in a post cataract surgery hyperopic refractive surprise. Conversely, in hyperopic LASIK, the central corneal power is steeper than pre-LASIK and a myopic refractive surprise may occur. Numerous formulas and methods have been applied clinically, such as the clinical history method, contact lens over refraction, and the Masket, Shammas and Haigis-L formulae, to name just a few, but each has its own methodology. Cataract surgeons typically compare a few formulae and often select the average, which can be time-consuming.

Things became theoretically simpler with the introduction of intraocular wavefront aberrometry, potentially bypassing formula-based calculations.

Intraoperative aberrometry, a term describing the use of a wavefront device during cataract surgery, has been available in the United States since 2008. Optiwave refractive analysis, (ORA, Alcon, Ft. Worth, TX) has been used in the United States since 2011. The ORA device uses a wavefront analysis of the eye, including both anterior and posterior effects of the cornea, during surgery at the point when the cataract has been removed. The information obtained is then transferred into a computer that can provide the proper power for the IOL.

ORA has been proven to provide more accurate IOL selection than commonly used preoperative IOL calculation formulas, not only in unusual cataract patients, such as those with axial length longer than 25 mm,[2] but also in postrefractive surgery cases with prior LASIK and PRK.[3,4,5]

5.10.5 If You Do Not Have an Intraoperative Aberrometer

Not all cataract surgeons have ORA or HOLOS (Clarity Medical Systems, Pleasanton, CA) devices available. Even if one routinely uses intraoperative aberrometry on patients with a history of previous corneal refractive surgery, we still highly recommend that several preoperative IOL calculations be performed for each patient. Which formula to use? With a total of 104 eyes with a history of previous myopic LASIK/PRK and subsequent cataract surgery, comparison among OCT-based formula, Barrett True K, Wang-Koch-Maloney, Shammas, Haigis-L, the conclusion of that study was "The OCT-based and the (Barrett) True K formulas are promising formulas."[6]

Other comparative peer reviewed studies also seem to favor the Barrett no history True K formula in this special group. It is at least as accurate as, or better than, commonly used formulas available on the ASCRS website (www.iolcalc.ascrs.org): in hyperopic LASIK/PRK,[7] in myopic LASIK/PRK,[8] and in RK.[9]

5.10.6 Special Challenges and Concerns for Patients with History of RK

Allow Enough Time between Surgeries on the Two Eyes until the First Eye Has Achieved a Stable Refraction

This becomes more important for RK than LASIK patients because the corneal LASIK flap incision typically does not change radically after cataract surgery. In contrast, with RK, swelling of the cornea incisions, immediately after cataract surgery, can flatten the cornea resulting in significant hyperopia. After a few weeks or so the immediate postop hyperopia tends to regress. Do not be confused between the immediate postoperative hyperopic change and the secondary slow and long duration hyperopic drift that occurs with RK patients. The second phase of hyperopic drift is the reason why we add extra myopic power, not the first phase.

Wait for 2 to 3 months for the refraction of the operated eye to stabilize before making a decision for the fellow eye. We typical select a target of -0.75D to account for the expected long term hyperopic drift if the cornea has four to six cuts, -1.00D if eight cuts. With more than 8 cuts, such as 12 or 16 cuts, we typical do not believe patients are good candidates for IOL monovision.

Limitations of Intraoperative Aberrometry

Unlike patients with a previous history of LASIK and PRK, the validation of ORA in patients with a history of radial keratotomy (RK) has not been well studied in the peer reviewed literature.[5] ORA has been, however, widely used among cataract surgeons on patients with a history of RK but the structural changes after LASIK/PRK versus RK are quite different. As we know, IOP can be up to 80 to 90 mm Hg during phacoemulsification, which may make the weak cornea change shape or even open the cuts in severe cases. The corneal shape and curvature at a pressure of 21 mm Hg just prior to the ORA reading may be quite different from the preoperative measurements. Because of this acute change, it is also possible to have subsequent changes in anterior chamber depth and axial length, based on which, ORA provides recommendations for the IOL power. Further studies are needed to establish validation. We recommend that surgeons be cautious when using ORA on RK patients, especially for those who have more than four cuts.

A Case Report

A 57-year-old man had been followed at F. Z.'s office since 1999 for his mild background diabetic retinopathy (BDR), moderate cataract, and status post RK in 1985. At his office visit in 2016, he wanted to have cataract surgery due to progressive driving and reading difficulty.

Preoperative Examination

Corrected distance vision
OD 20/30 with + 7.75 + 0.25 × 151;
OS 20/30 with + 6.00 + 0.50 × 132
His corneas had eight RK cuts in each eye and one astigmatic keratotomy cut OS.

IOP was 17 mm Hg each eye (Average IOP for the last 17 years between 1999 and 2016 was calculated and it was also: OD 17 OS 17.)
Corneal topography
OD 33.22/34.53 @135;
OS 34.51/36.76 @58
Preoperative refractive targets and IOL power with the Barrett True K formula:
OD -1.25 with + 32.00 SN60AT
OS -1.50 with + 30.00 SN60AT
No IOL monovision was offered due to longstanding significant diurnal fluctuation of his vision. Monovision does not work well in this situation.

Surgery was performed OS with a 2.4 mm incision aiming for -1.50 D. Four aphakic readings were taken and ORA recommendations were + 26.00 to + 26.50 (aiming for -1.43 D). Because of a 3.50 D discrepancy between the preoperative calculation and ORA recommendation, a + 27.50 D SN60AT IOL was used.

At 2-week follow-up, the patient was very happy. Distance vision OS was 20/30 + 2 with -1.50 + 1.00 × 070 in his left eye. He was eager to have right eye surgery done sooner rather than wait 2 to 3 months because of the significant anisometropia and his preplanned summer vacation. Right eye surgery was done aiming for -1.25 D. Four aphakic readings were taken. The ORA recommended + 25.50D for -1.25D, but + 26.50 was used due to the preoperative recommendation from the Barrett True K formula 32D aiming at -1.25 D. Two weeks after the second eye surgery, his distance vision OD was 20/25 with + 4.50 sphere and OS 20/25 with + 3.25 + 1.00 × 151. Observation was advised since the hyperopia could be attributed to early postoperative hyperopic drift. Macular OCT OU showed no macular edema to count for his hyperopic refraction. At the 3-month follow-up, his distance vision was OD 20/30 with + 1.75 + 1.50 × 089; OS 20/25 with + 0.50 + 0.75 × 055. He declined a piggyback IOL for OD. If there had been no adjustment the IOL choice IOL by 1 D in each eye, the postoperative hyperopia would have been worse.

A thorough review of the preoperative biometry showed no errors in the calculations. The case was subsequently reviewed by Alcon's ORA team, but the etiology for the unexpected hyperopic outcome could not be identified. Intraoperative K readings were not retrievable.

Not All RK Patients Are Good Candidates for IOL Monovision

Most patients with LASIK/PRK do well with IOL monovision and some even do well with multifocal and EDOF IOLs, but RK patients are often the opposite. It is our anecdotal experience that RK patients with very significant diurnal vision fluctuation, or with more than 8 cuts are not great candidates for IOL monovision, especially in bilateral RK patients.

5.10.7 Summary: Monovision Pearls for Previous Refractive Surgery Patients

Cataract patients with a history of previous corneal refractive surgery usually do well with IOL monovision, but with a few exceptions. Preoperative consultation is very important for clarification of reasonable expectations. If they had previously achieved refractive surgery induced monovision, it is advisable to keep the same pattern in terms of conventional vs. crossed IOL monovision regardless of the preoperative eye dominance test. Intraoperative aberrometry, such as ORA, has been demonstrated to improve the refractive outcomes of patients with LASIK/PRK, but its validation in RK patients still requires more studies. Recent peer reviewed comparison studies seem to favor the Barrett no history True K formula in the selection of IOL power for patients with a history of myopic LASIK/PRK, RK, and hyperopic LASIK/PRK.

References

[1] Lundström M, Barry P, Henry Y, Rosen P, Stenevi U. Evidence-based guidelines for cataract surgery: guidelines based on data in the European Registry of Quality Outcomes for Cataract and Refractive Surgery database. J Cataract Refract Surg. 2012; 38(6):1086–1093

[2] Hill DC, Sudhakar S, Hill CS, et al. Intraoperative aberrometry versus preoperative biometry for intraocular lens power selection in axial myopia. J Cataract Refract Surg. 2017; 43(4): 505–510

[3] Ianchulev T, Hoffer KJ, Yoo SH, et al. Intraoperative refractive biometry for predicting intraocular lens power calculation after prior myopic refractive surgery. Ophthalmology. 2014; 121(1):56 60

[4] Fram NR, Masket S, Wang L. Comparison of intraoperative aberrometry, OCT-based IOL formula, Haigis-L, and Masket formulae for IOL power calculation after laser vision correction. Ophthalmology. 2015; 122(6):1096–1101

[5] Canto AP, Chhadva P, Cabot F, et al. Comparison of IOL power calculation methods and intraoperative wavefront aberrometer in eyes after refractive surgery. J Refract Surg. 2013; 29(7): 484–489

[6] Wang L, Tang M, Huang D, Weikert MP, Koch DD. Comparison of newer intraocular lens power calculation methods for eyes after corneal refractive surgery. Ophthalmology. 2015; 122(12): 2443–2449

[7] Hamill EB, Wang L, Chopra HK, Hill W, Koch DD. Intraocular lens power calculations in eyes with previous hyperopic laser in situ keratomileusis or photorefractive keratectomy. J Cataract Refract Surg. 2017; 43(2):189–194

[8] Abulafia A, Hill WE, Koch DD, Wang L, Barrett GD. Accuracy of the Barrett True-K formula for intraocular lens power prediction after laser in situ keratomileusis or photorefractive keratectomy for myopia. J Cataract Refract Surg. 2016; 42(3): 363–369

[9] Ma JX, Tang M, Wang L, Weikert MP, Huang D, Koch DD. Comparison of newer IOL power calculation methods for eyes with previous radial keratotomy. Invest Ophthalmol Vis Sci. 2016; 57(9):OCT162–OCT168

6 Special Situations

Abstract

Monovision correction shows promise as an alternative treatment for patients with longstanding symptomatic but stable secondary diplopia. This may be accomplished with contact lenses or intraocular lenses (IOLs), if conventional management fails to promote fusion function. This approach should be considered with caution. More female than male patients choose laser vision correction monovision. Age does not seem to have a major impact on IOL monovision. Patients with a successful history of contact lens or laser vision correction monovision are almost universally good candidates for IOL monovision and the same pattern should be kept regardless of the dominant eye test. Patients with large pupils are probably less favorable for IOL monovision for nighttime driving. Pseudophakic monovision does not seem to have a negative impact on peripheral vision. Just like hand and foot sidedness, more people have their right eye as their sighting dominant eye than their left eye. Pseudophakic monovision may have a short period of adaptation, but no known study exists on this subject. When needed, non-customized over-the-counter readers seem to work quite well for most mini and modest level anisometropic IOL monovision patients.

Keywords: monovision to correct diplopia, gender and IOL monovision, age and IOL monovision, pupil size and IOL monovision, sidedness of ocular dominance, peripheral field and monovision, over-the-counter readers and IOL monovision

6.1 Monovision to Correct Diplopia

Some studies have shown a unique function of monovision as a means to correct symptomatic diplopia.[1,2,3,4] The principle of this approach is based on further suppression from monovision-induced anisometropia to dampen diplopia awareness. For nondiplopic presbyopic patients, we use monovision to increase depth of focus by binocular summation and monocular blur suppression. Therefore, we try to avoid those who have any history of strabismus, diplopia, or prism correction because we do not want to interrupt and compromise the existing balanced binocular function if they are currently not diplopic. However, for those

patients who are already diplopic with stable strabismus, which is the main clinical problem for these patients, we can use monovision to further disassociate the two eyes, while retaining a good field of vision, monocular acuity, and gross peripheral stereopsis.

Bujak et al[1] did a prospective study with 20 presbyopic patients (older than 45 years) who had symptomatic diplopia due to secondary strabismus with a deviation angle of 10 prism diopters or less and were stable for at least 3 months. Mean duration of diplopia was 44.3 months, ranging from 6 to 96 months. Subjects were excluded if they were not presbyopic or if they were satisfied with their previous prism correction for their diplopia. Each received monovision spectacles, contact lenses, or both, with distance correction in the dominant eye, as determined by the hole-in-card test. Half received a +3.00-diopter add and the other half received +2.50 diopters. Based on the results of the Diplopia Questionnaire, 85% of patients experienced significant improvement in diplopia symptoms after monovision correction. The quality of life score also increased significantly. There was improved social contact and appearance ($p = 0.0002$) with increased self-confidence resulting from personal appearance. There was no significant difference between the 2.50 D group and 3.00 D group. In spite of the advantages and benefits of purposeful monovision with either glasses or contact lenses, or both, the study did demonstrate some associated problems from this approach, such as difficulty in estimating distance, checking driving blind spots, and climbing or descending stairs.

Another study reported seven cases of diplopic patients successfully treated with contact lens monovision.[2] The author made the recommendation to instruct the patient not to think about which eye was seeing at which distance. Instead, encourage the patient to view the target of regard clearly. Prescribing distance correction for the less mobile eye also helped overall performance.

Extreme intraocular lens (IOL) monovision with 3.00 D or more anisometropia (9 out of 12 had 3.00 diopters or more and the remaining 3 had 2.00 to 3.00 diopters) was reported by Osher et al[4] to be successful in managing longstanding stable secondary diplopia in 12 patients. Those patients demonstrated the elimination or significantly decreased awareness of preoperative diplopia and achieved significant spectacle independence and high postoperative satisfaction. All the patients were warned of a possibility of surgical reversal if that new extreme IOL monovision should fail for any reason. All 12 cases attained excellent uncorrected distance vision and uncorrected near vision. There were no surgical reversals or postoperative prisms needed for any patient. No patient reported being dissatisfied. This is certainly an interesting and novel approach for longstanding stable secondary diplopia in patients with bilateral visually significant cataracts.

6.2 Other Factors Affecting Monovision

6.2.1 Gender

A number of laser vision correction studies demonstrate that slightly more women chose monovision than men.[5,6,7,8] The cosmetic aspects could be one motivation. No data are known demonstrating whether one gender has greater success with monovision.

6.2.2 Age

A literature review consisting of 26 known successful monovision patients and another 26 known unsuccessful monovision patients showed the mean age between the two groups was not statistically different.[9] It is our anecdotal impression that in IOL monovision, older patients tend to have greater satisfaction than younger patients, but we could not make a meaningful comparison because the number of unsatisfied patients is very small and most IOL monovision patients are elderly. That also seems to explain why it is more common to use preoperative contact lens trials for younger laser vision correction monovision when it is rarely needed for older IOL monovision cataract patients.

6.2.3 Previous Experience

Those who have a history of happiness with contact lens monovision or natural monovision are almost universally great candidates for IOL monovision. Of note, for those patients, it is better to keep the same pattern as before, regardless of the dominance test result. A similar phenomenon was noted in laser vision–induced monovision: "Every monovision contact lens wearer chose monovision correction over bilateral distance vision."[5] This phenomenon indirectly tells us the attraction and beauty of monovision. Once experienced and adapted to, the overwhelming majority of patients would like to keep it rather than reverse it or choose another modality.

6.2.4 Pupil Size

Patients with small pupils seem to do better with IOL monovision, especially for nighttime driving, likely due to the impact of depth of focus.[10,11]

An experimental study by Schor et al[12] of contact lens wearers demonstrated that pupil size is one of the very important factors for monovision function in scotopic conditions such as nighttime driving. Patients with small pupils had better interocular suppression than those with larger pupils. The study had only four monovision patients, but that conclusion is consistent with our own clinical experience, although it differs from what was noted in the study by Collins and Goode.[13]

6.2.5 Peripheral Field

Monovision has no adverse effect on the peripheral visual field.[9,14]

In monovision, although one eye is focused for far and the fellow eye focused for near, they both maintain good peripheral fields. Why is there no diplopia or visual confusion? It is most likely due to automatic foveal suppression[15,16,17,18] while the rest of the retinal image is still contributing to binocular function. The suppression of image blur happens mainly in the central 2 to 3 degrees of the visual field.[15] It is totally different from monocular occlusion.

6.2.6 Sidedness

Most people are clearly aware of which hand they favor to throw a ball, or which foot to kick a soccer ball, but eye dominance is not that clear, although we do have a favored eye for sighting. It has been suggested that these asymmetries are linked to the specialization of the left hemisphere of the brain for language, speech, and motor control. In humans, these biases are all rightward: handedness about 90%, footedness about 80%, and eyedness about 70%.[19]

More people have their right eye as their sighting dominant eye than their left eye. An experimental study with Parson's nonoptoscope, which is similar to the hole-in-card test, by Kommerell et al[20] found roughly two-thirds of studied subjects have a right sighting dominant eye and one-third have the left eye as the sighting dominant eye. Hillemans did a study with the pointing-a-finger method as the dominance eye test in which he found right ocular dominance in 40% of patients, left ocular dominance in 20% of patients, and uncertainty in 40%.[20] A study done by Lopes-Ferreira et al[21] noted the right eye was dominant in 70.5% by sighting dominance on the hole-in-card test and 61.4% by sensory + 1.50 D lens testing in 44 healthy presbyopic patients.

6.2.7 Adaptation

Up to 3 weeks are often necessary for monovision adaptation. [1,9,14,22] Harris and associates[22] observed an improvement in stereoacuity from 151 seconds to 90 seconds of arc after 3 weeks of monovision contact lens correction. Change in blur suppression with time was noted to be small, so adaptation in monovision is probably not very important.[9] Collins and colleagues found that during the first 8 weeks of contact lens monovision, patients had noticeable improvement in walking and hand–eye coordination.[23] There is no known study on this subject with IOL monovision, although it does not seem to be an issue in clinical practice.

There is no known study of IOL monovision regarding adaptation. Mini and modest IOL monovision patients seemed to be able to appreciate improved functionality immediately without a period of neuroadaptation, which is necessary in some patients with multifocal IOLs.[24]

A study by Fawcett et al[25] on 32 longstanding (6 months or longer) laser vision corrected monovision patients and 20 age-matched control adults demonstrated that binocular vision recovery may not happen immediately after the near vision eye is corrected for distance. That study suggested two possibilities: (1) binocular function in adults is not hardwired but rather continues to be susceptible to change throughout life; (2) the full binocular function cannot be immediately reversed by providing full binocular vision correction in those longstanding monovision adults. Our clinical experience with IOL monovision seems to confirm very satisfying binocular function once patients put on backup glasses, although we are not aware of any study similar to Fawcett et al's study in patients with IOL monovision with backup glasses or contact lens. (See detailed discussion in the section "Decreased Stereovision" in Chapter 7.)

Over-the-Counter Readers

It is our anecdotal experience that for mini and modest IOL monovision, over-the-counter reading glasses work well for the vast majority of patients if there is no significant astigmatism in either eye. For full monovision, customized readers may be needed should the patient need further assistance in prolonged reading, regardless of coexisting cylinder. We are not aware of any study on this subject.

References

[1] Bujak MC, Leung AK, Kisilevsky M, Margolin E. Monovision correction for small-angle diplopia. Am J Ophthalmol. 2012; 154(3):586–592.e2

[2] London R. Monovision correction for diplopia. J Am Optom Assoc. 1987; 58(7):568–570

[3] Migneco MK. Alleviating vertical diplopia through contact lenses without the use of prism. Eye Contact Lens. 2008; 34(5): 297–298

[4] Osher RH, Golnik KC, Barrett G, Shimizu K. Intentional extreme anisometropic pseudophakic monovision: new approach to the cataract patient with longstanding diplopia. J Cataract Refract Surg. 2012; 38(8):1346–1351

[5] Braun EH, Lee J, Steinert RF. Monovision in LASIK. Ophthalmology. 2008; 115(7):1196–1202

[6] Jain S, Ou R, Azar DT. Monovision outcomes in presbyopic individuals after refractive surgery. Ophthalmology. 2001; 108(8):1430–1433

[7] Goldberg DB. Laser in situ keratomileusis monovision. J Cataract Refract Surg. 2001; 27(9):1449–1455

[8] Wright KW, Guemes A, Kapadia MS, Wilson SE. Binocular function and patient satisfaction after monovision induced by myopic photorefractive keratectomy. J Cataract Refract Surg. 1999; 25(2):177–182

[9] Jain S, Arora I, Azar DT. Success of monovision in presbyopes: review of the literature and potential applications to refractive surgery. Surv Ophthalmol. 1996; 40(6):491–499

[10] Kawamorita T, Uozato H, Handa T, Ito M, Shimizu K. Effect of pupil size on visual acuity in a laboratory model of pseudophakic monovision. J Refract Surg. 2010; 26(5):378–380

[11] McDonald JE, Deitz D. Neuroadaptation to Monovision. In: Chang DF, ed. Mastering Refractive IOLs: The Art and Science. Thorofare, NJ: Slack Incorporated; 2008:295–301

[12] Schor C, Landsman L, Erickson P. Ocular dominance and the interocular suppression of blur in monovision. Am J Optom Physiol Opt. 1987; 64(10):723–730

[13] Collins MJ, Goode A. Interocular blur suppression and monovision. Acta Ophthalmol (Copenh). 1994; 72(3):376–380

[14] Ambati BK, Strauss L, Azar DT. Preoperative optical considerations in LASIK: refractive errors, monovision, and contrast sensitivity. In: Azar DT, Koch DD, eds. LASIK: Fundamental, Surgical Techniques, and Complications. New York, NY: Marcel Dekker; 2003:101–110

[15] Key JE, Rigel LE. Monovision Guidelines for Success. Continuing Education for Optometrists & Opticians. Elkins Park, PA: Pennsylvania College of Optometry; 1994 [sponsored by Johnson & Johnson Vision Products, Inc.]

[16] Evans BJ. Monovision: a review. Ophthalmic Physiol Opt. 2007; 27(5):417–439

[17] Simpson T. The suppression effect of simulated anisometropia. Ophthalmic Physiol Opt. 1991; 11(4):350–358

[18] Humphriss D. The psychological septum. An investigation into its function. Am J Optom Physiol Opt. 1982; 59(8): 639–641

[19] Carey DP. Vision research: losing sight of eye dominance. Curr Biol. 2001; 11(20):R828–R830

[20] Kommerell G, Schmitt C, Kromeier M, Bach M. Ocular prevalence versus ocular dominance. Vision Res. 2003; 43(12): 1397–1403

[21] Lopes-Ferreira D, Neves H, Queiros A, et al. Ocular dominance and visual function testing. Hindawi Publishing Corporation, BioMed Research International. Volume 2013, Article ID 238943. 7 pages http://dx.doi.org/10.1155/2013/238943

[22] Harris MG, Sheedy JE, Gan CM. Vision and task performance with monovision and diffractive bifocal contact lenses. Optom Vis Sci. 1992; 69(8):609–614

[23] Collins M, Bruce A, Thompson B. Adaptation to monovision. Int Contact Lens Clin. 1994; 21:218–224

[24] Barrett GD. Monovision with monofocal IOLs. In: Chang DF, ed. Mastering Refractive IOLs: The Art and Science. Thorofare, NJ: Slack Incorporated; 2008:440–453

[25] Fawcett SL, Herman WK, Alfieri CD, Castleberry KA, Parks MM, Birch EE. Stereoacuity and foveal fusion in adults with long-standing surgical monovision. J AAPOS. 2001; 5(6): 342–347

7 Limitations of Pseudophakic Monovision

Abstract

Pseudophakic monovision does have downsides, such as decreased fine stereopsis and contrast, although the impact in real life is very mild. These disadvantages increase as the anisometropic level increases. Monovision occasionally can induce diplopia in patients who have a history of double vision, prism use, extraocular muscle surgery, amblyopia, or monofixation syndrome. This situation happens more frequently if crossed rather than conventional intraocular lens (IOL) monovision is applied. In these induced diplopia patients, either optical correction with glasses or contact lenses, or surgical reversal can be successful to eliminate the symptoms. IOL monovision should not be viewed as a universal solution for presbyopia, but rather as an option available to carefully selected patients who do not have contraindications. Monovision is not recommended for pilots. Full monovision should be avoided for professional truck drivers, professional golfers, and baseball players, although mini-monovision seems to be very safe. Preoperative consultation and discussion of the possible need for glasses for nighttime driving is necessary. About two-thirds of monovision patients do not need glasses, but one-third still need to wear glasses for nighttime driving, either all the time or as back up.

Keywords: decreased stereopsis and IOL monovision, contrast and IOL monovision, monovision and induced diplopia, nighttime driving and IOL monovision, occupation and IOL monovision

7.1 Decreased Stereovision

Wheatstone[1] was believed to be the first to explain stereopsis, in 1838: "... the mind perceives an object of three dimensions by means of the two dissimilar pictures projected by it on the retina." Because each eye views the visual world from slightly different horizontal positions, each eye's image differs from the other, forming horizontal disparity, or binocular disparity. Wheatstone showed that this was an effective depth cue by creating the illusion of depth from flat pictures that differed only in horizontal disparity. To display his pictures separately to the two eyes, Wheatstone invented the stereoscope, which is still used today.

A review of contact lens and laser vision correction monovision by Jain et al[2] noted that stereopsis in monovision ranged from 23 to 73 arc seconds for distance, and 50 to 113 arc seconds for near, with a mean of 87.5 for near. Unsuccessful monovision had 50 to 62 arc seconds reduction in stereopsis compared with successful monovision patients. The presbyopic population was noted to have a significant decrease in stereopsis tested with the Titmus test with near correction when compared with the prepresbyopic population, but no difference was noted between males and females.[3] Another study, with 60 normal subjects aged 17 to 83 years, demonstrated that overall stereoacuity measured by all tests, including TNO and Titmus, showed a mild decline with age, and a significant drop off after age 50 with the Titmus test.[4]

Stereovision decreases when anisometropia increases.[5,6,7,8,9] A study by Fawcett et al[6] of 32 adults with LASIK/PRK-created monovision and 20 age-matched controls, with more than 6 months of follow-up, demonstrated a negative impact on stereovision and sensory fusion due to longstanding induced monovision. The monovision patients were divided into two subgroups based on anisometropic level: < 1.50 D as the low anisometropia group ($n = 18$) and 1.50 D or greater as the moderate group ($n = 14$). For the monovision study group patients, a single contact lens was used to correct the near eye for distance vision of 20/20 or greater at 6 m and then reading glasses were used to achieve vision of 20/20 or greater at 33 cm for reading. With this binocular full correction, a Randot stereovision test was performed at near and Worth Four Dot fusion test at 33 cm for extramacular sensory fusion and at far (3 m) for macular sensory fusion. These tests were done *within* 15 to 20 minutes of contact lens placement. A statistically significant difference was noted when the study groups were compared with the control group: the median stereovision was 100 seconds of arc for the low anisometropic group, 150 seconds of arc for the moderate anisometropic group, and 40 seconds of arc for control subjects. For foveal fusion tested with the Worth Four Dot test at 3 m, all control subjects passed the test.

Among patients with moderate anisometropia, 50% failed ($p = 0.009$). Among the low anisometropia group, 22% failed ($p = 0.182$). All subjects, both study and control patients, passed the extrafoveal Worth Four Dot test at 33 cm. This study not only suggested the impact of anisometropia level on stereovision and binocularity, but also suggested the susceptibility of fusion function in adults. Compromised binocularity may not recover immediately (within 15–20 minutes) even with full correction of anisometropia. The nature of binocularity can be plastic and the recovery may take longer. It would be very interesting if the same test were done again at 1 week and 3 weeks to compare with the results from the 15- to 20-minute test. Then, we would be able to tell if surgically induced longstanding monovision (at least 6 months in this study) has any permanent impact on stereovision and fusion, as well as how long the readaptation would take. No known study is available on intraocular lens (IOL) monovision in this regard. We routinely assume that backup glasses or contact lenses can fully recover binocularity immediately, but the real impact with accurate laboratory measurement is yet to be determined.

A study by Zhang et al[10] noted that average stereopsis was 127 seconds of arc when the average anisometropia was 1.93 D in 22 IOL monovision patients. The impact of IOL monovision on stereopsis was noted to be minimal when mini-monovision was applied.[11] A study by Goldberg[12] of 432 consecutive LASIK patients (51% full distance vision correction, 49% monovision correction with anisometropic levels following the age-based anisometropia Goldberg monogram[12]) noted almost identical results from their survey between the two groups in terms of depth perception.

There is no doubt that monovision has a negative impact on fine stereopsis, but when it comes to gross depth perception in normal activities of daily life, the negative effect is minimal. Our own 10-year IOL monovision review with a de-identified survey noted that 94.3% had no problem or pretty much no problem; 5.2% consider "it does not bother me even when I do not wear glasses"; and only 0.5% had to wear glasses all the time to correct their depth perception problem. (See details in the section "What Benefits Can Pseudophakic Monovision Bring to Your Practice?" in Chapter 1.)

7.2 Induced Diplopia

Contact lens–induced monovision can induce some esophoric shift (from exophoria to orthophoria or

to less exophoria, from orthophoria to esophoria or from less esophoria to more esophoria), but usually it is very small, averaging 1 to 3 prism diopters.[13,14] No effect was noted on vertical alignment.

Occasionally, monovision can cause diplopia and induce strabismus if contraindications are not excluded. Sometimes, a well-compensated ocular condition such as convergence insufficiency, accommodative esodeviation, intermittent exotropia, congenital fourth nerve palsy, and monofixation can deteriorate and cause manifest diplopia once IOL monovision is added. It may not be easy to recognize these problems when they are asymptomatic. For example, convergence insufficiency may show normal alignment at distance but exodeviation at near. If we check ocular alignment only at distance, we can easily miss this disorder. As we know, convergence insufficiency is quite common and typically worsens with age. Another example is monofixation syndrome. Because some monofixaters are orthophoric, especially those with primary monofixation syndrome with no known preceding ocular pathology, trying to avoid any tropic or > 8 to 10 diopter phoric patients for IOL monovision may not be enough, because one-third of monofixation patients show orthophoria on the cover and uncover test.[15] Intermittent strabismus can also be missed during a busy office eye examination. Intermittent strabismus itself, which allows partial bifixation, is not enough to cause permanent bifixation loss. Basically, those originally compensated asymptomatic patients can become symptomatic when the IOL monovision further weakens their fusion.

Pollard et al[16] studied 12 monovision-induced strabismus patients who had the onset of strabismus or recurrence of strabismus after obtaining monovision via contact lenses, LASIK, and cataract surgery with posterior chamber IOLs. Three of them had IOL monovision and the rest were contact lens–, LASIK-, or RK-induced monovision. All patients were first treated by converting the near eye to distance vision and then using reading glasses for near work. Seven regained fusion and five required surgery to reestablish motor or sensory control. The authors advised consideration of modest monovision, which has a smaller chance of disturbing binocularity, rather than a full monovision approach.

Kushner[17] reported 16 cases of acquired diplopia in patients who had a history of strabismus since childhood. In 6 of the 16 patients, monovision was the etiology due to a switched fixing eye. The induced diplopia disappeared in all these 16 fixation switch diplopia cases when proper optical correction was instituted to encourage fixation with the dominant eye.

Pratt-Johnson and Tillson[18] reported 24 cases of unilateral longstanding traumatic cataract from 1984 to 1988. All 24 cases had unilateral traumatic cataract and had intractable diplopia after their vision was restored with an IOL or contact lenses to vision of 20/40 or better. None of these cases had a known history of interrupted binocular function prior to their trauma and the average age at the trauma was 18 years. The study noted that the risk of diplopia increased if the interval from cataract formation to vision restoration was 2.5 years or longer. They also noted that these patients typically had secondary strabismus in the injured eye 1 year or longer after the injury. Compromised central fusion capability was believed to be the etiology.

Crossed monovision can sometimes cause problems if a long-suppressed eye becomes the distance fixating eye, such as in monofixation syndrome and unrecognized amblyopia, as in our cases reported in Chapter 4, in the section "Potential Contraindications and Concerns for Pseudophakic Monovision." When the longstanding suppressed eye becomes the fixating eye, whether surgically induced or spontaneously developed from cataract-induced refractive change, it may cause "fixation switch diplopia."[17,19] History taking is very important before we make a decision to offer IOL monovision. Generally, crossed IOL monovision works as well as conventional IOL monovision,[20,21] but caution should be used to avoid choosing the long-suppressed eye, or an amblyopic eye as the far vision eye for fixation. From another point of view, choosing the weaker eye for near vision with myopic defocus did not seem to cause major issues, although theoretically the extra burden of added anisometropia is unfavorable to maintaining asymptomatic extraocular muscle (EOM) balance. The binocular visual stress created by monovision can potentially cause esophoric shifts and these shifts are greater when the nondominant eye is corrected for distance.[22]

Induced diplopia is the main concern in IOL monovision. Overwhelmingly, we can do very well with IOL monovision if contraindications are avoided and the anisometropia is at a reasonable level. Anisometropia can have some impact on the extraocular muscle system, but it is typically very small, only an average of 0.6 to 0.9 prism diopter esophoric shift at distance was seen with monovision.[2,13] The esophoric shift in successful monovision was 0 to 0.6 D, much less than the amount of shift in unsuccessful monovision patients (2.1–2.2 D). The preoperative history cannot be overvalued to ensure that patients do not have compromised binocularity, such as diplopia, prism use, amblyopia, and EOM surgery. It is critical to check preoperative ocular alignment, preferably when the pupils are not dilated. If suspicion of monofixation or amblyopia exists, Titmus stereopsis, 4 diopters base out prism test, and Worth Four Dot tests are indicated. For very dense cataracts with very poor vision, the value and accuracy of these tests are limited or they are impossible to conduct, but for most cataract patients in developed countries, this is not common. We routinely check Worth Four Dot and Titmus stereopsis preoperatively for each surgical cataract patient if we are considering monovision. We have found this to be very helpful.

7.3 Compromised Contrast

The contrast sensitivity function increases by a factor of the square root of 2 ($\sqrt{2}$), or about 42%, when the stimulus is viewed binocularly rather than monocularly because of binocular summation.[2,23] Monovision mainly affects high spatial frequency contrast sensitivity,[7,23,24] but as the anisometropia increases to more than 1.50 D, the entire frequency range decreases and binocular summation is decreased significantly.[23,24]

In photopic illumination (e.g., $250\,cd/m^2$), monovision correction had no effect on visual acuity for both high and low contrast targets, but under low illumination, monovision patients may have some difficulty. This experimental result echoes our clinical impression that patients with IOL monovision are more likely to need backup glasses for nighttime driving.

During nighttime driving, the contrast between targets such as headlights of cars and a dark background can be challenging for monovision patients. Blur suppression does not work as well in scotopic and mesopic environments as in photopic environments, although successful monovision subjects still do better in suppressing blur at high contrast than unsuccessful monovision patients.[22,25] The contrast between bright objects and the background is much higher under scotopic than photopic conditions. The size of the object being viewed also has an impact on blur suppression. Smaller objects, such as an oncoming car headlight at night, make it more difficult for monovision patients to suppress blur.[25]

In low luminance, as the target contrast is lowered, the blurred image from the defocused eye is easier to suppress. As the contrast increases, it becomes more difficult to suppress the blur and the defocused image shows up as a halo.[26]

The anisometropic level in monovision can also affect the impact of contrast sensitivity. Contrast sensitivity decreases more as myopic defocus increases, mainly when it exceeds 1.50 diopters.[7,23,24,27,28]

7.4 Occupation Selection

It should be rare for the clinician to miss what the patient's visual goals and motivation for the consideration of monovision are, especially their main activities and hobbies. Because of the unique features of monovision, no matter whether corrected with spectacles, contact lenses, corneal laser procedures, or pseudophakic monovision, the practitioner has to remember to ask the patient about their occupation and avocations. In a medical-legal case[29] involving an airplane accident related to a contact lens monovision pilot, the practitioner was not aware of the occupation of the patient. According to the Federal Aviation Administration's Guide for Aviation Medical Examiners, the use of monovision contact lenses is not considered acceptable for aviation duty.[29] No known data exist to suggest a rate of higher motor vehicle accidents in monovision patients.[30]

It is also reasonable to avoid full IOL monovision for truck drivers, professional golfers, and baseball players. For truck drivers, our typical goal for the IOL refractive target is dominant eye plano to −0.25D and nondominant eye −0.50 to −0.75 D as mini-monovision, which works very well. The slightly myopic defocus will provide them better vision for the dashboard, computer, and cell phone. Anecdotally, we have not had unhappy patients in this setting. Full monovision at 1.75 D or more anisometropia should be avoided unless they are willing to wear glasses for nighttime driving.

7.5 Nighttime Driving

As discussed earlier, in photopic illumination, monovision correction has almost no detrimental effect on visual function for both high and low contrast targets, but under low illumination, monovision patients may have some difficulty.[7,22, 25,26] The contrast between bright objects and their background is much higher under scotopic than photopic conditions. Blur suppression does not sufficiently function in patients with strong ocular dominance. Even in patients with weak ocular dominance, under mesopic conditions in which the target appears highly contrasted with the background, blur suppression does not sufficiently function. Therefore, full monovision surgery is not recommended in patients whose occupation involves precise operations under low illumination or nighttime driving.

It is important to advise each IOL monovision candidate prior to cataract surgery that it may be necessary to wear glasses or contact lenses after cataract surgery for nighttime driving. Our 10-year IOL monovision review showed that about one-third of patients needed glasses for nighttime driving and two-thirds did not need glasses at all: about 65% of patients did not need glasses, 17% needed glasses for nighttime driving only in bad weather or heavy traffic, 16% needed glasses all the time for nighttime driving regardless of weather or traffic, and 2% did not drive any more due to vision concerns. The relatively high percentage of patients needing backup glasses for nighttime driving did not seem to affect their satisfaction because it was fully discussed before the cataract surgery: among all the de-identified surveys, 97% liked or really liked monovision, 2% were neutral, and 1% did not like it. (See details in the section "What Benefits Can Pseudophakic Monovision Bring to Your Practice?" in Chapter 1.)

References

[1] Wheatstone C. Contributions to the physiology of vision.–part the first. On some remarkable, and hitherto unobserved, phenomena of binocular vision. Philos Trans R Soc Lond. 1838; 128:371–394

[2] Jain S, Arora I, Azar DT. Success of monovision in presbyopes: review of the literature and potential applications to refractive surgery. Surv Ophthalmol. 1996; 40(6):491–499

[3] Emmes AB. A statistical study of clinical scores obtained in the Wirt stereopsis test. Am J Optom Arch Am Acad Optom. 1961; 38:398–400

[4] Garnham L, Sloper JJ. Effect of age on adult stereoacuity as measured by different types of stereotest. Br J Ophthalmol. 2006; 90(1):91–95

[5] Weakley DR. The association between anisometropia, amblyopia, and binocularity in the absence of strabismus. Trans Am Ophthalmol Soc. 1999; 97:987–1021

[6] Fawcett SL, Herman WK, Alfieri CD, Castleberry KA, Parks MM, Birch EE. Stereoacuity and foveal fusion in adults with long-standing surgical monovision. J AAPOS. 2001; 5(6): 342–347

[7] Johannsdottir KR, Stelmach LB. Monovision: a review of the scientific literature. Optom Vis Sci. 2001; 78(9):646–651

[8] Erickson P, McGill EC. Role of visual acuity, stereoacuity, and ocular dominance in monovision patient success. Optom Vis Sci. 1992; 69(10):761–764

[9] Lebow KA, Goldberg JB. Characteristic of binocular vision found for presbyopic patients wearing single vision contact lenses. [Review]. J Am Optom Assoc. 1975; 46(11): 1116–1123

[10] Zhang F, Sugar A, Jacobsen G, Collins M. Visual function and patient satisfaction: comparison between bilateral diffractive multifocal intraocular lenses and monovision pseudophakia. J Cataract Refract Surg. 2011; 37(3):446–453

[11] Labiris G, Giarmoukakis A, Patsiamanidi M, Papadopoulos Z, Kozobolis VP. Mini-monovision versus multifocal intraocular lens implantation. J Cataract Refract Surg. 2015; 41(1):53–57

[12] Goldberg DB. Laser in situ keratomileusis monovision. J Cataract Refract Surg. 2001; 27(9):1449–1455

[13] McGill EC, Erickson P. Sighting dominance and monovision distance binocular fusional ranges. J Am Optom Assoc. 1991; 62(10):738–742

[14] McLendon JH, Burcham JL, Pheiffer CH. Presbyopic patterns and single vision contact lenses II. South J Optom. 1968; 10: 7–10, 31, 36

[15] Parks MM. Th monofixation syndrome. Trans Am Ophthalmol Soc. 1969; 67:609–657

[16] Pollard ZF, Greenberg MF, Bordenca M, Elliott J, Hsu V. Strabismus precipitated by monovision. Am J Ophthalmol. 2011; 152(3):479–482.e1

[17] Kushner BJ. Fixation switch diplopia. Arch Ophthalmol. 1995; 113(7):896–899

[18] Pratt-Johnson JA, Tillson G. Intractable diplopia after vision restoration in unilateral cataract. Am J Ophthalmol. 1989; 107(1):23–26

[19] Boyd TAS, Karas Y, Budd GE, Wyatt HT. Fixation switch diplopia. Can J Ophthalmol. 1974; 9(3):310–315

[20] Zhang F, Sugar A, Arbisser L, Jacobsen G, Artico J. Crossed versus conventional pseudophakic monovision: Patient satisfaction, visual function, and spectacle independence. J Cataract Refract Surg. 2015; 41(9):1845–1854

[21] Kim J, Shin HJ, Kim HC, Shin KC. Comparison of conventional versus crossed monovision in pseudophakia. Br J Ophthalmol. 2015; 99(3):391–395

[22] Ambati BK, Strauss L, Azar DT. Preoperative optical considerations in LASIK: refractive errors, monovision, and contrast sensitivity. In: Azar DT, Koch DD, eds. LASIK Fundamental, Surgical Techniques, and Complications. New York, NY: Marcel Dekker; 2003:101–110

[23] Loshin DS, Loshin MS, Comer G. Binocular summation with monovision contact lens correction for presbyopia. Int Cont Lens Clin. 1982; 9(3):161–165

[24] Pardhan S, Gilchrist J. The effect of monocular defocus on binocular contrast sensitivity. Ophthalmic Physiol Opt. 1990; 10(1):33–36

[25] Schor C, Landsman L, Erickson P. Ocular dominance and the interocular suppression of blur in monovision. Am J Optom Physiol Opt. 1987; 64(10):723–730

[26] Collins MJ, Goode A. Interocular blur suppression and monovision. Acta Ophthalmol (Copenh). 1994; 72(3):376–380

[27] Hayashi K, Ogawa S, Manabe S, Yoshimura K. Binocular visual function of modified pseudophakic monovision. Am J Ophthalmol. 2015; 159(2):232–240

[28] Zheleznyak L, Sabesan R, Oh JS, MacRae S, Yoon G. Modified monovision with spherical aberration to improve presbyopic through-focus visual performance. Invest Ophthalmol Vis Sci. 2013; 54(5):3157–3165

[29] Nakagawara VB, Véronneau SJ. Monovision contact lens use in the aviation environment: a report of a contact lens-related aircraft accident. Optometry. 2000; 71(6):390–395

[30] Evans BJ. Monovision: a review. Ophthalmic Physiol Opt. 2007; 27(5):417–439

Index

Note: Page numbers set **bold** or *italic* indicate headings or figures, respectively.